Cognitive Remediation for Psyc

✓**Treatments** *That Work*™

Cognitive Remediation for Psychological Disorders

Therapist Guide

Alice Medalia • Nadine Revheim • Tiffany Herlands

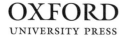
OXFORD
UNIVERSITY PRESS

2009

OXFORD
UNIVERSITY PRESS

Oxford University Press, Inc., publishes works that further
Oxford University's objective of excellence
in research, scholarship, and education.

Oxford   New York
Auckland   Cape Town   Dar es Salaam   Hong Kong   Karachi
Kuala Lumpur   Madrid   Melbourne   Mexico City   Nairobi
New Delhi   Shanghai   Taipei   Toronto

With offices in
Argentina   Austria   Brazil   Chile   Czech Republic   France   Greece
Guatemala   Hungary   Italy   Japan   Poland   Portugal   Singapore
South Korea   Switzerland   Thailand   Turkey   Ukraine   Vietnam

Published by Oxford University Press, Inc.
198 Madison Avenue, New York, New York 10016

www.oup.com

Oxford is a registered trademark of Oxford University Press

Library of Congress Cataloging-in-Publication Data
Medalia, Alice.
Cognitive remediation for psychological disorders : therapist guide /
Alice Medalia, Nadine Revheim, Tiffany Herlands.
p.   cm.
Includes bibliographical references.
ISBN 978-0-19-538371-3
1. Cognitive disorders—Patients—Rehabilitation.   I. Revheim,
Nadine.   II. Herlands, Tiffany.   III. Title.
RC553.C64M43 2009
616.89'1425—dc22

                                                    2008043838

9 8 7 6 5 4 3 2 1

Printed in the United States of America
on acid-free paper

About Treatments *ThatWork*™

Stunning developments in healthcare have taken place over the last several years, but many of our widely accepted interventions and strategies in mental health and behavioral medicine have been brought into question by research evidence as not only lacking benefit, but perhaps, inducing harm. Other strategies have been proven effective using the best current standards of evidence, resulting in broad-based recommendations to make these practices more available to the public. Several recent developments are behind this revolution. First, we have arrived at a much deeper understanding of pathology, both psychological and physical, which has led to the development of new, more precisely targeted interventions. Second, our research methodologies have improved substantially, such that we have reduced threats to internal and external validity, making the outcomes more directly applicable to clinical situations. Third, governments around the world and healthcare systems and policymakers have decided that the quality of care should improve, that it should be evidence based, and that it is in the public's interest to ensure that this happens (Barlow, 2004; Institute of Medicine, 2001).

Of course, the major stumbling block for clinicians everywhere is the accessibility of newly developed evidence-based psychological interventions. Workshops and books can go only so far in acquainting responsible and conscientious practitioners with the latest behavioral healthcare practices and their applicability to individual patients. This new series, Treatments *ThatWork*™, is devoted to communicating these exciting new interventions to clinicians on the frontlines of practice.

The manuals and workbooks in this series contain step-by-step detailed procedures for assessing and treating specific problems and diagnoses. But this series also goes beyond the books and manuals by providing ancillary materials that will approximate the supervisory process in assisting practitioners in the implementation of these procedures in their practice.

In our emerging healthcare system, the growing consensus is that evidence-based practice offers the most responsible course of action for the mental health professional. All behavioral healthcare clinicians deeply desire to provide the best possible care for their patients. In this series, our aim is to close the dissemination and information gap and make that possible.

This guide teaches clinicians and therapists how to set up and run a cognitive remediation program for clients who are cognitively impaired. Cognition in this context refers to functions such as attention, memory, abstract reasoning, and visual spatial analysis.

Because chronic mental disorders are often associated with cognitive deficits, the program described can be helpful for those individuals suffering from cognitive deficits associated with schizophrenia, affective spectrum disorders (depression and bipolar disorder), and alcohol and substance abuse. The Neuropsychological and Educational Approach to Cognitive Remediation (NEAR) is a group-based treatment with proven efficacy that provides individualized learning to participants. Clients meet at least twice a week for 60–90 minutes and use computers and educational software to work on their specific areas of impairment. At the end of each session, clients participate in group discussion.

This guide provides detailed information for the cognitive remediation specialist (CRS) on setting up a "learning center," stocking a software library, recruiting clients, performing intakes and assessments, creating treatment plans, and dealing with difficult clinical situations. It includes all the materials you need to run a successful program.

David H. Barlow, Editor-in-Chief,
Treatments *ThatWork*™
Boston, MA

References

Barlow, D. H. (2004). Psychological treatments. *American Psychologist, 59*, 869–878.

Institute of Medicine. (2001). *Crossing the quality chasm: A new health system for the 21st century*. Washington, DC: National Academy Press.

Contents

Chapter 1   Introductory Information for Therapists   *1*

Chapter 2   Treatment Principles   *7*

Chapter 3   Setting Up a Cognitive Remediation Program   *25*

Chapter 4   Selecting Appropriate Software   *43*

Chapter 5   Intake and Assessment   *61*

Chapter 6   Treatment Planning   *71*

Chapter 7   Strategies for Treating Specific Cognitive Deficits   *85*

Chapter 8   Phases of Treatment   *95*

Chapter 9   Bridging Groups   *109*

Chapter 10   Dealing With Difficult Clinical Situations   *129*

Chapter 11   Program Evaluation   *139*

Appendix   *145*

References   *159*

About the Authors   *163*

Chapter 1   *Introductory Information for Therapists*

What Is Cognitive Remediation?

Cognitive remediation is a behavioral treatment for people who are experiencing cognitive impairments that interfere with daily functioning. Cognition refers to a broad set of abilities that together allow us to perceive, process, manipulate, and respond to information. Examples of cognitive functions are attention, memory, abstract reasoning, and visual spatial analysis. Although the term *remediation* sometimes implies that the cognitive skill was once better and has since declined, this is not necessarily the case. It is possible that the skill never developed adequately, even though the potential was once there. Cognitive remediation is different from standard education in that it focuses on the underlying cognitive skills and not on developing domain-specific knowledge, such as science or arithmetic. It is also not intended to teach people how to read or write because that is best done with literacy techniques. Cognitive remediation is intended to help people develop the underlying cognitive skills that will make them better able to function in daily tasks, including those performed in school, work, social interactions, and independent living. For example, it might help someone become more attentive so that he can better focus on schoolwork, household tasks, or job responsibilities. Cognitive remediation is intended for individuals who are experiencing problems in specific areas of cognition.

From a psychiatric rehabilitation perspective, cognitive remediation is considered one of the skill-training interventions. Like other psychiatric rehabilitation interventions, it focuses on skills and supports in order to improve the success and satisfaction people experience in their chosen living, learning, working, and social environments. Because individuals are more likely to achieve goals they have chosen, the specific cognitive skill and support interventions used are based on the individual's self selected overall rehabilitation goals. Like other psychiatric rehabilitation interventions, cognitive remediation is a collaborative process of assessing a person's skills and supports related to his goals, planning with the person how to enhance his skills and supports, and intervening to develop the skills and/or supports needed to achieve the person's goals (Anthony et al., 2002).

Why Provide Cognitive Remediation to Psychiatric Patients?

Severe Psychiatric Illness Is Frequently Associated With Cognitive Deficits

Impairments in attention, memory, processing speed, and problem-solving ability are the most common cognitive deficits found in patients with schizophrenia, depression, bipolar disorder, and alcohol and substance abuse. The severity and profile of these deficits vary depending on factors like diagnosis, course of illness, and social-environmental factors. In schizophrenia, a generalized cognitive decline is evident early on in the illness, with superimposed relatively greater problems in attention, memory, processing speed, and problem solving (Gold & Harvey, 1993). Patients with psychotic illnesses typically score below 85% of the general population on cognitive tests. These cognitive deficits are persistent and not simply related to an episode of illness. Thus, even when a person is psychiatrically stable, cognitive impairment remains evident.

Medication does not have a major impact on cognitive impairment in schizophrenia. There appears to be a positive impact on the gross attentional problems associated with acute psychotic decompensation, but the enduring attentional problems that are seen throughout the course of the illness are surprisingly resistant to medication (Cornblatt, Obuchowski, Schnur, & O'Brien, 1997; Keefe et al., 2007). In the affective disorders, medication can significantly reduce attention problems if attentional deficits are state related and the illness responds to psychopharmacologic intervention. In treatment-refractory patients, attentional problems tend to persist (Glahn et al., 2007). Furthermore, some medications used to treat affective disorders can impair attention. When medications are not in therapeutic range, or are idiosyncratically tolerated, they can cause cognitive impairment.

Cognitive Deficits Are Associated With Poor Outcome

Impairments in attention, memory, and problem solving have been associated with functional outcome in psychiatric patients (Bowie et al., 2008). In schizophrenia, impaired cognition has consistently been associated with poor social problem solving and difficulty benefiting from rehabilitation services (Green, 1996; Green, Kern, Braff, & Mintz, 2000). Psychosocial skills training is a form of rehabilitation that is widely available for people with persistent psychiatric illness, and it is intended to teach basic life skills like social interacting, illness management, independent living, and leisure skills (Silverstein, 2000). Patients who have more severe attentional problems are least likely to acquire skills in these programs. The attentional problems make it difficult for them to process the information given in groups, and they may not be able to sustain attention for the duration of the sessions (Spaulding et al., 1999).

Cognitive deficits make it difficult to succeed at work (McGurk & Meltzer, 2001). If your ability to pay attention and remember information is worse than 85% of the other people applying for a job, you are at a distinct disadvantage. Most jobs require people to multitask and prioritize information. For example, a cashier must be able to ring up the items, answer questions, remember information about sales, and deal with coupons. It can be very difficult to perform well at work if you have trouble attending to and remembering information.

Cognitive deficits make it difficult to manage independent living (Velligan, Bow-Thomas, Mahurin, Miller, & Halgunseth, 2000). Many clients with attention and memory problems struggle with things like remembering their keys, remembering where they put important items, and remembering appointments. People with problem-solving deficits have trouble organizing their living space so that they can find things, may have trouble maintaining a budget, find it difficult to negotiate public transportation, and may be prone to making unwise decisions and judgments.

Cognitive Deficits Increase the Risk for Psychiatric Decompensation

Psychiatric decompensation is thought to occur because of an interaction between vulnerability factors and stress factors. Vulnerability factors are those factors that exist within the person, perhaps biologically or genetically determined, that give the person a predisposition for developing a psychiatric illness. Stress refers to conditions that are experienced as overwhelming or unmanageable. Cognitive impairment acts in both ways. Some cognitive deficits like attention impairment are evident during and between episodes of active psychosis and have been noted in individuals at risk for schizophrenia. Attention impairment is therefore considered to be a trait or vulnerability marker of schizophrenia. It is thought to be one critical link in the chain of events that cause psychosis. Other cognitive deficits are not vulnerability factors but cause stress, which in turn contributes to decompensation. Take, for example, the depressed person whose memory problems are interfering with job performance to the point that his employer is threatening termination. That causes considerable stress, low self-esteem, and anxiety, which in turn may precipitate psychiatric decompensation. If treatment focuses only on the emotional problems, the cognitive problems will persist and there will be greater risk of poor outcome.

Cognitive impairments can also impact psychiatric stability through their direct and indirect effects on motivation. Someone with deficits in working memory (the ability to hold information in mind while considering it) may have difficulty holding in mind the steps to reach a goal, even a valued goal like submitting a job application or completing home or school projects. Unable to negotiate the task at hand, the person may not engage in valued behaviors and without the practice may fail to develop competencies. In turn, the self-perception of incompetence demotivates the person and keeps him from initiating valued behaviors like job seeking. Cognitive deficits, like poor memory or attention, may also render someone more dependent on others to manage tasks and in turn leave the person feeling ineffectual. When people feel ineffectual and incompetent, they are less likely to maintain a recovery-oriented focus, and that will impact psychiatric stability.

When Should Cognitive Remediation Be Provided to Psychiatric Patients?

Cognitive remediation should be provided when it is apparent that cognitive deficits are interfering with functional outcome. It can be provided to children, adolescents, and adults. In the younger populations the treatment may be thought of as cognitive enhancing or rehabilitative because the brain and cognitive skills are still developing. Cognitive remediation is a service that is best provided once the person is stabilized from acute decompensation. That is not to say that there is no role for cognitive remediation on acute services. Assessment and initial treatment is possible and has been shown to be effective in this setting. However, with length of stay on acute care units decreasing so dramatically, it is difficult to have sufficient time for cognitive remediation. Cognitive remediation is best done within the context of a rehabilitation-oriented program so that it is possible to integrate the goals of cognitive remediation with the overall rehabilitation goals.

Where Should Cognitive Remediation Be Provided?

Cognitive remediation is typically provided in community-based programs and long-term-care settings. It is best done within the context of a rehabilitation program because the rehabilitation model focuses on skills training. Rehabilitation psychology emphasizes an integrated approach to the patient which appreciates the complex interaction of cognitive, emotional, and environmental variables in the recovery process. From this perspective, cognitive deficits are not seen simply as a manifestation of brain dysfunction, but rather social-cognitive dysfunction. Rehabilitation programs focus on skills development and seek to give patients the tools to function adaptively and independently in society. Cognitive remediation provides one set of tools that allows for the cognitive as well as social-emotional needs of the patient to be addressed. Together, cognitive remediation and the other rehabilitation services promote a smooth interplay of cognitive and emotional variables in everyday functioning.

What Is It Like to Have Cognitive Impairments?

Imagine that you want to get your high school diploma but every time you sit in class your mind wanders and you cannot pay attention. Your teacher becomes critical and other students ridicule you or resent you for holding the class back. You try to learn the material, but your memory is poor. As hard as you try, you fail the tests. After a while, you start to feel stupid. You may give up and decide it is better not to try than to keep failing. You may think that work will be easier than school. You get hired, but quickly anger the boss when you forget to do something. People speak rapidly and ask you to do several things, leaving it unclear what is the most important thing, what to do first. You get overwhelmed and anxious, and get nothing done. You are worried that if you ask for help you will be criticized. It is not easy having a cognitive deficit. You look normal. You are not in a cast or wheelchair, so people do not see that there is a problem and become helpful. Everyone else seems to move and work more quickly and with ease, and you start to feel incompetent. That feeling of incompetence makes you doubt your ability to handle situations. When we feel incompetent we are unhappy with ourselves and sometimes angry at others. In contrast, when we feel competent we feel content and able to take control of our lives.

Cognitive remediation can provide a bridge to self-efficacy and empowerment by breaking the cyclical downward spiral of feeling incompetent and "giving up." As people experience success at tasks that require attention and memory, problem solving, and processing speed, they begin to see themselves as competent to complete the various tasks they set for themselves in everyday life. Thus, cognitive remediation not only enhances cognitive skills, it also provides an experience of success and thereby empowers the person to feel competent to tackle valued goals. As such, cognitive remediation can be an important step in the recovery process.

Chapter 2   *Treatment Principles*

Every treatment approach is guided by certain beliefs, has certain goals, and is based upon a theoretical foundation that informs the interventions and procedures used. In the first chapter, we discussed the rationale for doing cognitive remediation with psychiatric patients. This chapter will focus on the theoretical foundation and goals that inform the Neuropsychological Educational Approach to Cognitive Remediation (NEAR). NEAR is a method of cognitive remediation that we developed for psychiatric patients. It is a group-based treatment that provides highly individualized learning, by allowing each person in the group to work at her own pace on tasks carefully chosen both to be engaging and to address her cognitive needs. NEAR has been successfully implemented in a variety of settings ranging from inpatient care, to outpatient rehabilitation programs, to supportive housing facilities, schools, and forensic settings (Medalia & Freilich, 2008).

The Goals of NEAR

1. To improve those neuropsychological (cognitive) functions identified as sufficiently impaired to hamper functional outcome.

2. To provide a positive learning experience to each and every client.

3. To promote independent learning skills.

4. To promote a positive attitude about learning.

5. To promote awareness about learning style, and learning strengths and weaknesses.

6. To promote a sense of competence and confidence in one's ability to acquire skills.

7. To promote awareness of how social-emotional context affects cognitive functioning.

8. To promote optimal cognitive functioning in different social contexts.

It is important to note that these goals are highly interrelated. For example, we do not believe that much improvement in cognitive functions will occur unless the person develops self-awareness, a sense of competence, and a positive attitude about learning. Likewise, we do not think that there is much value in improving a cognitive skill without appreciating the social-emotional context in which it is used. Finally, the ultimate goal of NEAR is for the client to be an independent learner, to not need the program, and to be able to continue the learning process in mainstream educational, vocational, and social settings.

Overview of NEAR Program Structure

In general, NEAR is conducted in groups of six to eight clients. Not only is group treatment more effective from an administrative standpoint, it also has therapeutic advantages. In a group, a sense of community often develops among the clients because they share the same highly valued activities of learning and self-improvement. This sense of relatedness among group members satisfies an important psychological need and promotes increased motivation and task engagement. Furthermore, in a group there are also opportunities for peer leadership.

Although the NEAR session is a group in the sense that there are several people in the room, it differs from most group therapies because each person works at her own pace on tasks chosen to address her particular needs. Clients can work together if they want, but do not have to, a situation that is ideal for people who struggle with social interactions. Because clients work at their own rate, there is a rolling admission to the groups. It is not administratively or clinically advantageous to wait to start a group until all six people have been interviewed. Rather, the groups slowly develop as the clinician enrolls more people. Should one client then leave, another one is recruited to fill the spot. This way, groups are composed of clients in different stages of treatment, and those who have progressed farther can help the newly enrolled ones. This benefits both the veteran participant who assumes a mentor role and the new client who has a peer role model.

Clients participate in NEAR sessions at least twice a week, and the sessions are typically 60–90 min long. About two thirds of the time involves individual cognitive activities, usually on the computer, and a third of the time is spent in a bridging group, which is a verbal group for all the participants to discuss how the individual activities relate to real-world situations. When clients enter NEAR sessions, they first work on the computer, choosing exercises from the list of software shown to them by the clinician. Everyone has a folder that details the software exercises she has been shown by the clinician. On any given session, the client can choose to work on any task from that list.

As important as the software is to the NEAR program, it is not the defining feature. A common misconception is that exposing clients to the educational software used in NEAR will improve cognition. This misses the essential element of NEAR—that it is a theory-based therapeutic approach. Each session is structured to enhance motivation and learning through a set of carefully implemented instructional techniques. It is the clinician's job to learn these instructional techniques so that she can more effectively administer the therapy.

Snapshot of a NEAR Session

NEAR sessions look deceptively simple to run. The visitor will see clients waiting outside the door for the session to start. They come into a room, quietly pick up their work folders, choose a software program from a box of disks, sit down at a computer, and start up their chosen activity. The clinician is there, perhaps greeting people, perhaps reminding someone that today she will show them a new activity, or perhaps just sitting at a table watching the whole process. Each client works at her own pace on programs that she has chosen to work on—programs chosen from the list of activities she has been shown how to use by the clinician or peer leader. If the client is working on a task that remediates basic cognitive skills like working memory or attention, the client will work on at least two tasks during the session. If the client is working on a complex task, she may stay on that task the whole session. Clients who have been attending the group for some weeks are highly focused and engaged in their work. Newer clients are less independent, work in a focused manner for briefer periods, and may require more staff intervention. Thirty minutes before the 90-min session ends, the clinician announces it is time for group discussion. Clients end their computer-based activities, take out their folders and write what they have done that day, and turn their chairs around and participate in a discussion about how their computer activities relate to things they do in everyday life. Participants share strategies for solving problems on the cognitive exercises and in real life.

The job of the clinician in NEAR sessions varies from assessing, to instructing, to observing. Much of the time clients work independently, but the clinician is always there, carefully but unobtrusively monitoring their progress, and ready to facilitate a more positive learning experience if there are indications that the client needs help or guidance. The clinician watches closely how clients perform tasks and considers what about their performance of the task indicates how they will be successful or unsuccessful in meeting their rehabilitation goals. Each session is intended to provide a positive learning experience, and the clinician intervenes as necessary to achieve this goal.

Theoretical Foundations

NEAR is eclectic in nature, drawing from numerous theories and helping strategies. The following sections discuss the theoretical foundations and influences that form its underpinnings.

Neuropsychological Influences

Neuropsychology and the related field of cognitive psychology have made major contributions to our understanding of both cognitive operations and the underlying neuronal basis for cognition. For example, the attention system is understood to comprise subsystems that perform different but interrelated cognitive functions. These different subsystems are mediated by different anatomic areas, which together work as a network. Sometimes neuropsychological functions are referred to as nonsocial cognitive functions in as much as they refer to pure cognitive functioning, or the basic cognitive processes that operate regardless of environmental context. The profile of cognitive impairment informs the intervention strategy. Those deficits that limit functional outcome and put the person at risk for decompensation are considered the important ones to target for intervention.

Cognitive impairment has long been the focus of treatment in programs for individuals with head injury, and many remediation exercises have been developed to improve cognitive deficits in that population. These exercises show the influence of neuropsychological models of cognition in their singular focus on specific nonsocial aspects of cognition. For example, in attention remediation, the ability to focus, encode, rapidly process and respond, maintain vigilance, and avoid distraction from competing stimuli are aspects of attention that may be isolated for remediation. Often these exercises are computerized to facilitate standardization of presentation, precise measurement of response, and provide frequent feedback.

Rehabilitation programs for individuals with head injury have identified different types of remediation strategies that are effective: Restorative, compensatory, and environmental manipulation. A restorative approach to cognitive remediation attempts to identify and directly repair impaired cognitive skills by using drill and practice exercises. Intervention approaches developed within the context of the restorative model typically remediate deficits in a stepwise, hierarchical progression, with attentional deficits addressed prior to remediation of higher-order deficits in problem solving or memory. Compensatory remediation techniques do not attempt to restore the impaired cognitive skill but rather to compensate for, or circumvent, the deficit with reliance on intact cognitive skills. Thus, someone with poor memory may be taught to use organizational strategies to rely upon when memory fails. Often, the first step in compensatory remediation is to make sure that the patient has sufficient awareness of her cognitive deficit to maintain the necessary motivation and interest in applying new compensatory techniques. We have found that in psychiatric patients a gradual process of building self-awareness is critical for laying the groundwork in teaching compensatory skills. Environmental manipulation refers to the changes in the environment that are made to facilitate optimal cognitive functioning. The use of organizers, calendars, and a key hook by the door are examples of environmental manipulations.

Neuropsychology provides a background for understanding the nature of the cognitive deficits we target, but it does not inform us about how skills are best learned and what factors influence recovery. It is in this regard that learning and educational theory, and rehabilitation psychology have a major influence.

Learning Theory and NEAR

The use of techniques like shaping, errorless learning, prompting, modeling, and frequent positive feedback reflect the influence of learning theory.

Errorless learning refers to the careful titration of difficulty level so that the client learns without resorting to trial and error, and has a positive experience with increasing challenge. The client is started at a level that is believed to be easy enough to guarantee success, and then the level of difficulty is slowly increased.

Shaping and positive feedback are other methods that have been found effective for treating cognitive impairment. Shaping is the process of systematically reinforcing an individual for demonstrating behaviors that increasingly approximate a target behavior. In NEAR, we use shaping to improve cognitive skills and to improve behaviors like punctuality, attendance, and staying on task. When we give clients weekly, and then, eventually, monthly certificates congratulating them for the number of times they attended sessions, we are shaping behavior with positive reinforcement. When the client is doing a problem solving exercise and receives praise for a good answer, her skills are being shaped.

Prompting is a technique that responds to the client's current difficulty in the learning exercise, not by explicitly providing correct information but, instead, by asking open-ended questions that guide the person toward the correct response. This promotes task engagement, self-competence, and an active learning style. If the therapist were to do the problem for the client, it would promote passivity.

Modeling, or demonstration of a solution, is occasionally necessary when prompting fails to guide the client toward a correct response. Modeling is only done in the context of an immediate goal, and should be brief and accompanied by succinct verbal explanation.

Generalization refers to the transfer of a learned skill or behavior to other situations besides the one where the training occurred. Learning theory has indicated some of the factors that promote generalization of skill. Within the remediation exercises, target behaviors need to be paired with multiple cues, ideally in various contexts, so that the behavior will be elicited in multiple settings. In attention training this occurs when the desired response is paired with auditory, visual, and social cues embedded in a variety of tasks. Clients who do multiple tasks that exercise their cognitive abilities are more likely to improve than those whose training is limited to repetitive execution of one task.

Bridging is another technique that promotes generalization. In bridging, explicit connections are made between the cognitive skills acquired during sessions and the application of these skills in everyday life. Group therapy can be useful in promoting bridging. Clients can be encouraged to talk about the ways in which the skills they are using to complete the software exercises are relevant to daily life. Chapter 9 provides more information on bridging.

Educational Psychology and NEAR

Educational psychology has made significant contributions to our understanding of how people learn, the conditions under which they learn optimally, and the best strategies for effective teaching. Educational psychology has proven that people learn the most, learn the fastest, and retain knowledge longest when they are excited and motivated to learn (Schunk, Pintrich, P. R., & Meece, 2007). This excitement about learning is called intrinsic motivation. Intrinsic motivation is the motivation to do an activity because performance of that activity is in and of itself rewarding. Intrinsic motivation is the inherent inclination to explore, learn, seek, challenge, and test one's abilities. This contrasts to extrinsic motivation, which occurs when there are external rewards for performing an action.

Intrinsic motivation has other benefits besides increasing learning. It is also associated with increased levels of autonomy, self-determination, and sense of well-being (Ryan & Deci, 2000). People who are intrinsically motivated to get well are more likely to adhere to treatment recommendations. There are a number of teaching techniques that promote intrinsic motivation and a positive attitude about learning. These techniques also increase learning, depth of engagement in a learning activity, and sense of competence. Because apathy, anhedonia, and avolition are frequent symptoms in the severely mentally ill, and these motivational problems compromise engagement in treatment, it is important to use teaching techniques that increase intrinsic motivation.

Intrinsic motivation and task engagement occur when tasks are contextualized, personalized, and allow for learner control (Cordova and Lepper, 1996). Contextualization means that rather than presenting material in the abstract, it is put in a context whereby the practical utility and link to everyday life activities are made obvious to the client. In attention remediation, a decontextualized focusing task would require the person to press a button every time a green square appears on the otherwise blank computer screen. A contextualized focusing task would require the person to assume the role of pedestrian in a task that simulated the experience of responding to a crosswalk signal.

Personalization refers to the tailoring of a learning activity to coincide with topics of high interest value for the client. For example, if the person likes to drive, she is more likely to enjoy a problem solving task that has her negotiating the challenges that arise when driving cross-country rather than doing a task that teaches the abstract principles of problem solving. Personalization also refers to the learner entering into the task as an identifiable and independent agent, for example, signing in by name or assuming a role (truck driver, detective, or trader) in a task that simulates a real-world activity. Learner control refers to the provision of choices within the learning activity, in order to foster self-determination. In memory training, this occurs when the client can choose task features like difficulty level or presence of additional auditory cues when doing a visual memory exercise.

Educational psychology has also provided research on the important role of multisensory presentation of material. This allows for multiple processing of the information to be learned and promotes better retention of material. Another technique is to give opportunities to actively use information and skills. People are less likely to improve their memory if you simply tell them memory techniques than if you give them many auditory, visual, and kinesthetic memory exercises where they can apply different mnemonic strategies.

Rehabilitation Psychology and NEAR

Rehabilitation psychology emphasizes an integrated approach to the patient, which appreciates the complex interaction of cognitive, emotional, and environmental variables in the recovery process. From this perspective, cognitive deficits are not seen simply as a manifestation of neuropsychological dysfunction, but rather social-cognitive dysfunction. Rehabilitation psychology favors a more interactive learning process approach to cognitive remediation over the formal didactic exercises used in a purely cognition-oriented program. This allows for the social-emotional as well as cognitive needs of the patient to be addressed and promotes a smooth interplay of cognitive and emotional variables in everyday functioning.

NEAR is not a comprehensive rehabilitation program. Rather, it is intended to be used within the context of a rehabilitation program that offers clients the educational, vocational, social, and independent living skills that they require. NEAR provides the focus on cognitive functioning, but it does so with an appreciation of the social-emotional context in which cognition functions.

Self-Determination Theory and NEAR

Self-determination theory (Ryan & Deci, 2000) provides an approach to personality and motivation that examines how the interplay of social-contextual conditions and innate psychological needs fosters constructive development, well-being, happiness, and optimal functioning. Self-determination literally refers to those factors that determine the outcome/development of the self. According to this theory, optimal development of the self occurs when people are intrinsically motivated, self-regulating, and when their basic psychological needs are met. The basic psychological needs are identified as competence, autonomy, and relatedness. When these basic psychological needs are met, people become more intrinsically motivated.

NEAR strives not only to help improve specific cognitive functions, but also to help each person be the best learner they can. Intrinsic motivation is recognized as essential for the learning process, both to make someone a good learner and to enhance effectiveness of the specific cognitive exercises. Educational psychology has indicated aspects of learning activities that promote intrinsic motivation, for example, contextualization, personalization, and choice. Self-determination theory indicates other ways to promote intrinsic motivation for learning, namely, by fostering positive experiences of relatedness through interactions with the clinician and other members of the group, by providing opportunities to gain a sense of competence, and by encouraging autonomous functioning in learning environments.

Client-Centered Therapy and NEAR

Carl Rogers is best known for his development of client-centered therapy and counseling techniques, but he also had much to say about education and group work. Rogers focused on the **relationship** between educator and student. As he once wrote, "The facilitation of significant learning rests upon certain attitudinal qualities that exist in the personal relationship between facilitator and learner" (Rogers, 1967). He referred to the teacher as a facilitator, reflecting a belief that enactive learning is more effective than direct teaching.

NEAR clinicians can use the guidelines Rogers developed as a model for relating to clients. He believed that the clinician's ability to feel and convey genuineness (realness), acceptance, and empathy are "core conditions" for facilitating learning (Rogers, 1951). According to this model, NEAR clinicians who are comfortable with themselves and enter into the role as a real person who has no need to present a facade will be better able to communicate and meet the client on a person-to-person basis. Furthermore, clinicians who value the client's feelings, learning style, and opinions, and can relate in a caring but nonpossessive way are likely to be successful at facilitating learning. Rogers wrote about prizing the learner as an imperfect and complex human being with many potentials, and he encouraged clinicians to have confidence and trust in the capacity of the human being to change and develop. He also wrote about the importance of teachers and clinicians being able to understand a student's reactions to the learning process without judging, a process he called empathetic understanding. In NEAR, the clinician uses this understanding to better guide the learning process and enhance the dialogue with the client about metacognition and her unique approach to learning. NEAR clinicians are also encouraged to view themselves as *facilitators* who create the environment for engagement in the learning process by having an attitude that fosters exploration and autonomy.

Computers and NEAR

Computers have been used for several decades within the educational system because they provide a platform on which to easily present learning exercises that incorporate the basic educational principles known to promote learning. It is possible to design educational software that provides multisensory feedback, gives frequent feedback and positive reinforcement, promotes success and builds confidence, gives the individual choice and the ability to control nonessential aspects of the learning process, and promotes a sense of joy in learning. With computerized exercises, difficulty levels can be individualized so that the task is challenging but not frustrating, and the client can be given ample opportunity to apply the targeted skill in contextualized formats. Computers also have the advantage over teachers of being able to very consistently provide objective feedback. Computers do not have a bad day and do not register fatigue or frustration when the client fails yet again; they are programmed to provide encouragement and positive feedback. Furthermore, clients enjoy working on computers because they are viewed as prestigious and are socially valued. Clients who engage in computer-mediated remediation often receive positive reinforcement from impressed friends and family.

The computer itself simply provides the overall learning platform; the software provides the learning tools. The design of the software program, and whether or not it incorporates basic educational principles, largely dictates whether the remediation experience will be frustrating or engaging. Computer exercises exert a remedial effect on cognition through two broad categories of mechanisms: specific and nonspecific. *Specific mechanisms* refer to those aspects of the activity that focus specifically on a cognitive function. The *nonspecific mechanisms* refer to those aspects of computer activity that promote or facilitate skill acquisition without directly targeting a specific cognitive skill. An example of a nonspecific mechanism would be the personalization that occurs when you type in your name and are greeted by name. Personalization is known to facilitate learning. Both specific and nonspecific mechanisms contribute meaningfully to the overall therapeutic effect.

Outcomes Research

We have had many years of clinical experience doing NEAR, and the improvements clinicians see in their clients, and the numerous expressions of enthusiasm the clients have voiced about their experiences, can be viewed as one indication of treatment success. Treatment outcomes research is another important way to test the efficacy of NEAR (Medalia & Richardson, 2005). The aim of this kind of research is to see if clients make gains in the program and if these gains carry over to real-life situations. A mixture of randomized controlled trials and community-based outcome studies have been used to examine this question, reflecting the need to study NEAR both in the laboratory and as it is used in daily practice. Some studies have looked at the effectiveness of various NEAR exercises, whereas other studies have looked at the impact of the program as a whole. The outcome measures typically include cognitive functioning, psychiatric status, and psychosocial functioning. Because the goal of cognitive remediation is to improve cognitive functioning and functional outcome, as opposed to training-task performance, we only consider studies where treatment efficacy has been defined as a change in cognition as measured by an independent test, or by evidence of functional change. Some of the measures of real-world functioning have included treatment compliance, independent living skills, psychosocial functioning, psychiatric status, and educational and occupational advancement.

Impact of NEAR on Cognitive Functions

A multisite randomized waitlist control trial of NEAR was conducted with 40 participants between the ages of 17 and 50, who carried a diagnosis of schizophrenia or schizoaffective disorder (Hodge et al., 2008). The immediate treatment group received 20–30 sessions of NEAR over 15 weeks, whereas the waitlist group waited 15 weeks before starting their 20–30 sessions of NEAR. Both groups received standard treatment as usual. Following treatment, significant improvements were found in the areas of attention, processing speed, executive functioning, and delayed verbal and visual memory. These gains were sustained 4 months after treatment ended.

Attention

One controlled study found that state-hospitalized patients with schizophrenia made significant improvement on the Continuous Performance Test (CPT) after 18 sessions of attention training (Medalia, Aluma, Tryon, & Merriam, 1998). Patients in the control group did not make significant change on the CPT on retest, but those given attention remediation did, and their improvement was significantly greater than that of the control group. The attention training given was called Orientation Remediation Module (ORM), a computer package that we now rarely use in NEAR because patients prefer the more visually engaging educational programs, which are also effective (Hodge et al., 2008).

Problem Solving

A controlled study of inpatients with chronic schizophrenia or schizoaffective disorder found beneficial effects for patients who worked on the software program Where in the USA is Carmen Sandiego?[®] The patients who received ten sessions of treatment made significantly more improvement on an outcome measure that assessed problem solving skills for independent living than patients who did not work on the Carmen Sandiego software. The outcome measure used in this study was The Independent Living Scale (ILS), a semistructured interview that assesses whether there are sufficient problem solving skills to make successful community living likely. It is noteworthy that significant change was seen after only 10 sessions of working on the software. Of further interest is the finding that subjects liked working on the Carmen Sandiego software and wanted to continue even after the study ended. This suggests that it was an intrinsically motivating activity for them (Medalia, Revheim, & Casey, 2001).

Another study examined whether the gains made by the patients in the previously discussed study persisted over a period of time. Patients who worked on the Carmen Sandiego software for 10 sessions were then retested on the ILS after 4 weeks of not receiving cognitive remediation. It was found that the gains made by the group exposed to problem solving remediation persisted 4 weeks later. The patients who did not receive problem solving remediation by working on the Carmen Sandiego software continued to show no gains on retest with the ILS. These results provide more evidence of the benefit of problem solving training techniques that promote intrinsic motivation and generic problem solving strategies (see Medalia, Revheim, & Casey, 2002).

In order to evaluate the effectiveness of short-term remediation with acutely ill patients, a randomized controlled study was done on an acute care psychiatric unit with a 14-day average length of stay. Some patients carried the diagnosis of schizophrenia, whereas others had an affective disorder. The treatment group was given 6 hours of exposure to the Carmen Sandiego software for improving problem solving skills, whereas the control group worked on Mavis Beacon Teaches Typing®, another software program that does not require problem solving. The patients who worked on Carmen Sandiego made significantly more improvement than the control patients on a test of verbal problem solving. This suggests that verbal problem solving deficits are responsive to short-term intervention in acutely ill patients (Medalia, Dorn, & Watras-Gans, 2000).

Memory

Memory deficits are notoriously difficult to treat, and most remediation efforts focus on compensatory strategies. In this study, inpatients with chronic schizophrenia or schizoaffective disorder were given two 25-min sessions a week for 5 weeks, during which time they worked on an engaging software program developed to improve memory skills. Patients in the control groups did not receive memory remediation. Despite the fact that patients receiving memory remediation improved on the remediation tasks themselves, this benefit did not carry over to an improvement on various memory tests given as an outcome measure. A possible reason for this failure in generalization is that the treatment was too focused and brief. A number of cognitive skills, such as attention and organizational strategies, facilitate optimal memory. Therefore, a more broad-based and comprehensive approach to remediation may be more likely to work (Medalia, Revheim, & Casey, 2000).

Indeed, the previously referenced multisite randomized controlled trial using the full NEAR program (Hodges et al., 2008) found that participants in 20–30 sessions of NEAR made significant change on measures of delayed verbal and nonverbal memory. These clients had been exposed to a number of different software programs discussed in this manual, and thus had been given an opportunity to develop their skills in attention, processing speed, working memory, organization, problem solving, as well as memory. Thus, it seems more likely that memory will improve if a broad-based cognitive remediation program is implemented.

Processing Speed and Reaction Time

There is evidence from a community-based outcome study that NEAR can lead to improvements in processing speed as used in a vocational task. Choi and Medalia (2005) followed 48 outpatients with schizophrenia and affective spectrum disorders who took the Minnesota Clerical Test (MCT) before and after 26 sessions of NEAR. The MCT is a clerical speed test that requires processing speed and sustained attention. Thus, it is both a proxy vocational functioning measure as well as a neurocognitive test. As a group, the 48 clients showed significant improvement on the MCT, indicating that 26 sessions of NEAR results in improvement in processing speed and sustained attention.

Reaction time refers to the visual motor response, and unlike measures of processing speed, the score does not take into account accuracy of response. Many clients are quite slow to respond to stimuli when they enter remediation, and considerable work needs to be done to encourage a faster response. The program Frogger is an example of a software exercise we sometimes use to increase reaction time. In the study of attention training mentioned earlier (Medalia et al., 1998), clients in the treatment group made significant improvement in reaction time over the course of 18 sessions. These clients had worked on the ORM, a series of attention training exercises, many of which have a reaction time component.

Impact of NEAR on Psychiatric Symptoms

Several randomized controlled treatment trials support a modest positive effect of NEAR on psychiatric symptoms. A study by Medalia, Dorn, et al. (2000) found that six sessions of NEAR exercises led to significant improvements on both a self-report measure of ability to cope with psychiatric symptoms and a rating of global psychopathology provided by nurses.

Another randomized controlled trial with chronically ill inpatients (Bark et al., 2003) reported that only the psychiatric inpatient group exposed to a brief 10-session course of problem solving training improved significantly over time on the Positive, Negative, and General Psychopathology Subscales of the Positive and Negative Symptoms Scale (PANSS). Between group differences were not significant.

The treatment-controlled study referenced in the studies of attention found that the inpatients with chronic schizophrenia who made significant improvements in attention also showed significantly more improvement on the Brief Psychiatric Rating Scale (BPRS) than the patients in the control, no cognitive remediation, condition (Medalia et al., 1998). The BPRS measures a range of psychotic and affective symptoms and consists of 18 symptom and behavior constructs, each rated on a seven-point scale of severity. It is used to assess treatment response of psychiatric patients in controlled clinical trials.

Impact of NEAR on Psychosocial Functioning

Several community-based outcome studies and one randomized controlled trial have examined the impact of NEAR on measures of psychosocial functioning. The previously referenced multisite randomized waitlist control trial (Hodge et al., 2008) found that participants exposed to 20–30 sessions of NEAR in 15 weeks duration made significant improvements on the Social and Occupational Functioning Assessment Scale (SOFAS).

Revheim, Kamnitzer, Casey, and Medalia (2001) examined outcomes of 87 mixed diagnosis outpatients enrolled in a NEAR program that was part of an Intensive Psychiatric Rehabilitation Treatment (IPRT) program. Using utilization as a reflection of treatment engagement, they found that of clients not engaged in NEAR, 60% attended their scheduled IPRT programs, whereas of clients who additionally received NEAR, 82% attended regularly scheduled treatment programs. Furthermore, 88% of IPRT clients who received NEAR completed all their IPRT goals, whereas of IPRT clients not receiving NEAR, only 5% completed all their IPRT goals. Rates of psychiatric hospitalization were 10% for NEAR participants and 22% for IPRT clients who did not attend

NEAR. These data suggest that participation in NEAR improves over-all treatment engagement, ability to accomplish treatment goals, and ability to avoid rehospitalization.

Medalia et al. (2003) in their outcomes study of 27 clients with severe and persistent mental illness, referred for NEAR from a supportive housing facility for the homeless, reported that after 6 months 52% of these clients enrolled in an educational program to get their GED and 22% started a vocational internship. None of these clients had previously been successfully engaged in vocational/educational services, suggest-ing that participation in the NEAR program facilitated advancement in functional outcome.

Choi and Medalia (2005) examined the pre- and posttreatment Work Behavior Inventory (WBI) scores of 48 outpatients with schizophre-nia and affective spectrum disorders exposed to 26 hours of NEAR. The WBI is a 34-item supervisor-rated scale that measures work-related behaviors that are essential for successful employment. In this study, subjects were found to have significantly improved work-related behav-iors, suggesting that attendance at NEAR can benefit work readiness behaviors.

Taken together, these studies indicate that participation in NEAR impacts not only cognitive skills, but psychosocial functioning as well.

Chapter 3 | *Setting Up a Cognitive Remediation Program*

Cognitive remediation programs function best within larger mental health rehabilitation programs. Like other psychiatric rehabilitation interventions, cognitive rehabilitation aims to improve the likelihood that people will experience success and satisfaction in their chosen living, learning, working, and social environments. When cognitive remediation is provided in the context of a rehabilitation program, it is easier to link the specific cognitive skill and support interventions to the individual's overall rehabilitation goals. Furthermore, when the clinician is secure in the knowledge that the other aspects of the client's care will be attended to, he can then focus on the task of improving cognition. In essence, a space is created where the patient and clinician can focus on cognition, knowing that even if major clinical problems are present, they will be addressed elsewhere. Much as employees are expected to focus on work during scheduled hours, and not bring in personal problems, we expect our clients to put other problems aside and focus on the job of improving their cognition. This can only be done if there is a comprehensive treatment plan in place that the cognitive remediation therapist, together with other clinicians, works to implement.

To have a cognitive remediation program, one needs clients, physical space, staff, time, start-up money, and the commitment and support of the rehabilitation program and administration. The specific features of each of these components are detailed in the sections that follow. It is essential that there is at least one person designated to run the cognitive remediation program and that he has the time allotted to do only that. In general, a staff commitment of 20 hours a week will suffice to handle a caseload of 36, assuming 6 clients are seen at a time. If a novice clinician is assigned to the program, then he will require ongoing weekly supervision with someone who is familiar with this treatment modality. As with any new program, administrative support is crucial. Valuable time can be wasted if equipment, supplies, and space issues are not expediently addressed.

The Setting

It is important to consider the setting of the cognitive remediation program because it impacts the nature of the client population, the goals, and the very essence of the work. Cognitive remediation programs can work in a large variety of settings: inpatient/outpatient, acute/long-term care, forensic, jails, school-based mental health programs, dual diagnosis, and substance abuse centers. Adaptations may need to be made to accommodate the overall structure of the larger setting, and the goals of the program may vary accordingly.

Equipment and Materials

Space is a prerequisite for program development, and in many settings this is a precious commodity. If six clients are going to be seen at a time, the program room should be at least 150 square feet. Larger rooms are better, but the room should not be so large that people feel lost in it. The space cannot be shared by other programs when clients are seen; there should not be other people using the space, or going in and out for any reason, when the program is in session. The room should be a calm place, without much visual distraction. A room overlooking a firehouse would, for example, be ill-advised. Windowless rooms are fine as long as there is adequate ventilation. The lighting should be good for reading and computer work. The furnishings should include either six-foot table(s) that accommodate two computers or separate computer stations. It is important that there be sufficient desk space around the computer to put papers. The clinician needs his own desk and computer, and a chair with wheels. Each computer station needs a chair of appropriate height for computer work. When working with adolescents, it is inadvisable to have them sit at rolling chairs. Other furnishings should include a locking file cabinet for the clinician to keep client files, a bookcase for computer software and books (alternatively, the software can be kept in one drawer of the file cabinet if it is a lateral file), and either a wall-mounted file holder or floor cabinet with slots for clients to keep their working files accessible. One bulletin board, computer disc containers, and a calendar will be needed. It is useful to have a map of the world displayed prominently on the wall, because geography is frequently a topic. Otherwise, there should not be much on the walls, which should be painted in light hues. Figure 3.1 is a photo of a well-designed Learning Center.

Purchasing Computers

As computers are a central part of the program, it is important to invest wisely in this piece of equipment. The computers have to be able to run the software, so it is helpful to know the software you will be using so that you can ensure hardware compatibility. Some software only runs off a disc and has auditory stimuli, necessitating a CD-ROM drive and

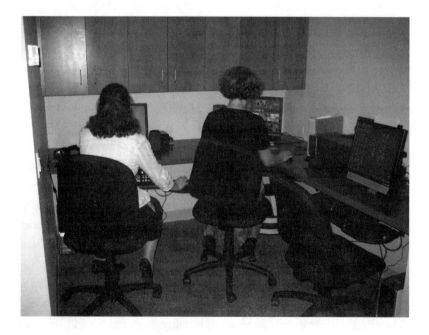

Figure 3.1
A well-designed Learning Center.

speakers. Most CD-ROM software may be hybrid and run equally well on Windows or Mac computers. The minimum central processing unit (CPU) requirements should include sufficient hard disk space for 20 programs because most programs require that some game components be installed on the hard drive and need sufficient processing speed to run programs effectively. Software-compatible video cards and speakers with compatible sound drivers are required. A color printer is needed; headphones are an attractive optional peripheral. Internet access is optional but useful to have on at least one computer. Larger monitors are easier to see, so we recommend 17-inch displays, although 15 inches is adequate. Purchasing hardware with the highest processing speed available and capacity to upgrade memory is a very valuable feature. With the rapid developments in computer technology, it is reasonable to assume that computers will have to be replaced and upgraded, but having adequate processing speed and the option to add memory can forestall that eventuality. Finally, it is possible to use laptops in situations where portability is an issue, although they are typically more expensive and should be purchased with a peripheral mouse, because the touch pads are difficult to use. A touch screen may also be a user-friendly accessory.

Starting a Software Library

You should purchase a minimum of 12 software titles containing at least 20 different exercises so that there will be a sufficient range of difficulty, content, and activity to meet the varied needs of the target population. Considerable thought should be put into these purchases, and the reader is referred to Chapter 4 for guidelines on how to make these decisions. In addition to the initial budget for software, an annual budget for upgrades and new purchases needs to be set aside. On average, about five new programs need to be purchased annually if one is simply to keep up with developments in the field. Obviously, if the program is expanding and must serve more clients, or more varied needs, the budget should be increased so that more software can be purchased. Many software titles can be purchased in bundled sets of 2, 5, or 10 discs, an option that may be appealing for large programs. Otherwise, having one or two copies of each title is usually sufficient, and the clinician will need to structure sessions to accommodate those times when more than one client wants to work on the same program.

Naming the Program

The name of the program should be inviting so that people will want to belong. Belonging promotes a sense of well-being and reinforces self-determination and intrinsic motivation. Clients will benefit more and learn more quickly if they readily want to join and feel eager to explore what the program has to offer. Terminology like "cognitive remediation" can be off-putting, since it is technical and mechanical sounding and implies that something is wrong with the people who attend. A name like "The Learning Center" is much more inviting and emphasizes an opportunity (learning) that is valued in society. In this manual we will refer to the program as The Learning Center.

Staff Training and Supervision

There are no schools that formally teach how to do cognitive remediation with psychiatric patients, and there is no one group of clinicians trained in this specialty. Psychologists and occupational therapists receive didactic and practicum training in highly related areas. Other mental health professionals also have relevant experiences and knowledge bases. At this point in time, cognitive remediation is a skill that is taught in workshops or by a supervisor, someone who has clinical remediation experience to pass on in a highly individualized learning format. Eventually, cognitive remediation may be taught in graduate school, but like therapy or teaching, it will always be a skill that is ultimately developed within the practicum context. There is a knowledge base that will facilitate the clinical work, but other factors such as personality and interpersonal skills of the clinician are equally important. To be highly organized but not rigid or controlling, to be interested and curious about how people learn, to be observant without being judgmental, and to be committed to helping others be as independent as possible are good traits for the cognitive rehabilitation specialist (CRS) to have. Some people are "born teachers" or "born listeners," qualities that are invaluable in this kind of work.

Certain basic guidelines can be used when recruiting a CRS. If the expectation is that the CRS is to eventually function independently, the educational standards should be set higher than if ongoing supervision is to be provided. In general, clinicians who will be expected to run the program should have at least a Master's degree. Formal education in clinical psychology gives a solid base of knowledge in normal and abnormal psychology and the treatments of psychiatric disorders. An understanding of the neuropsychology of psychiatric illnesses is quite helpful and indeed essential if the CRS is to relate the remediation in a meaningful way to the deficits. Formal training in special education and/or occupational therapy and practicum experience with psychiatric populations also provide the CRS with a highly relevant knowledge base. Occupational therapists have considerable skills in regard to rehabilitation of cognitive deficits, and they have traditionally applied these skills in work with head-injured populations.

The junior staff assisting at The Learning Center do not require such an extensive formal educational background. They can conduct individual and group sessions but typically require weekly supervision of their cases and considerable direction on treatment planning and implementation. A college degree and background working in mental health is essential. Training in education, teaching, or special education is quite useful. All clinicians need to have an orientation to wellness and rehabilitation models and to have a profound respect for people's ability to learn.

New training will be required before embarking on this type of work. Clinicians need to acquire knowledge about how people learn, the cognitive deficits common in the persistently mentally ill, and the ways these deficits impact on daily life. The theoretical basis for the work should be explained, and the interface between cognitive rehabilitation and other treatment modalities has to be understood. In addition to acquiring the relevant knowledge base, training in computer work must be gained. The CRS will need to spend several weeks getting familiar with software before starting to see clients. Although some knowledge of working with computers and an ability to run the software is essential, it is not necessary to be an expert. In fact, it is the wise clinician who knows the value of being able to model for clients, how to be gracefully ignorant, and how to go about learning new skills. Inevitably someone, perhaps one of the clients, will prove to have some computer expertise, and it usually gives that person considerable pleasure to assume the role of teacher. It is important to regularly set aside time for training in new software. The programs are complicated, and it requires time to become familiar with all the different ways they can be used to remediate cognition.

Particularly when a program is first set up, it is important to provide sufficient supervision with a senior specialist. An initial period of intensive training may last a week. The staff will need time to get oriented to the computers and software, the various intake and daily procedures, and the procedures and programs of the larger clinic. In addition to the training of the cognitive remediation staff, other staff members have to become familiar with the new treatment modality so that they can make appropriate referrals and have realistic expectations of the program for their patients. This can be accomplished by offering in-services and open houses where hands-on experiences are offered to the referring staff members. If there are vocational or supportive educational programs that will be linked to the cognitive rehabilitation program, the vocational and educational counselors or job supervisors may need to be trained in making assessments of cognitive skills. The phase of settling in can take several months, and ultimately it is over the course of the first year that the program will slowly become integrated with the other mental health services that the patients are receiving.

As in psychotherapy training, it is unrealistic to expect that after a week of cognitive rehabilitation training a clinician would be ready to deal with the problems that arise in doing the daily work. Weekly supervision should be provided until the CRS feels ready to be more independent. Supervision can then decrease in frequency, perhaps occurring every other week, and then monthly, until it is no longer needed at all. It can be extremely helpful for beginning clinicians to observe a senior clinician doing an intake and conducting sessions. Similarly, after watching a senior clinician devise a treatment plan and implement it, the beginner will feel more at ease with the process. Senior clinicians can also provide support in dealing with the inevitable "systems" issues that arise in larger clinic settings. In this regard, it is also important to have an ongoing dialogue with administrative staff, in the form of periodic meetings between the director of the larger service and the cognitive rehabilitation clinician. This way, a more seamless delivery of service can be assured.

Patient Selection

The Neuropsychological and Educational Approach to Cognitive Remediation (NEAR) cognitive rehabilitation program is intended for a select group of individuals. It is a large group of individuals with diverse problems, but nevertheless there are characteristics that define the group. The success of the program depends largely on the careful screening of clients so that the treatment is applied to the right set of problems and people. It is particularly important for the beginning clinician to be very circumspect about the problems he will take on. Once the clinician gains a high level of expertise, the client selection criteria may be more flexibly applied, but in the beginning the following criteria should be rigorously exercised.

1. Age between 13 and 65

2. Premorbid intelligence level estimated at borderline or greater (IQ > 70)

3. Reading level greater than or equal to fourth grade

4. No active substance or alcohol abuse

5. Postdetox at least 1 month

6. No traumatic head injury within the past 3 years

7. Sufficient psychiatric stability to sit for sessions

These rather basic criteria are rooted in experience, empirical outcome studies, and neuropsychological and developmental theory. It is possible to apply the basic principles of the rehabilitation program to other populations, for example, younger or older patients, but modifications would need to be made to the program. As it is, these criteria are quite broad, and there are subgroups within this broadly defined population whose needs must be accommodated by individualized treatment plans.

The rationale for using these criteria reflects a wish to maximize positive outcome. Children under the age of 13 learn differently from older populations and require specific instructional techniques. Adolescents also have specific learning needs but the modifications are less dramatic. Furthermore, it is already possible to see the devastating effects that psychiatric illness can have on the existing skills of adolescents. Studies repeatedly show that neuropsychological test scores of adolescents decline around the time of the first psychotic break of schizophrenia, and depression also is associated with lowering of scores. The upper age limit suggested also reflects developmental issues; however, in this case, the 65-year cutoff is an acknowledgment of the natural decline in skills that can accompany the aging process. There is some evidence that maintaining an active mind and engaging in cognitively challenging activities is important for the elderly, and it is therefore quite likely that cognitive rehabilitation could prove to be productive. However, the approach would need to be modified to fit the needs of the population. Discussion of those modifications is beyond the scope of this book.

The recommended IQ cutoff is frequently a surprise to people referring clients to the program. Reasoning that the program is intended for cognitively impaired individuals, clinicians may try to refer mentally retarded or severely developmentally delayed people. This is not an appropriate population, because their needs are quite different from those of patients who have the cognitive capacity to learn at a fairly normal rate. Mentally retarded patients have a generalized cognitive deficiency and require different teaching methods to facilitate optimum cognitive growth. They learn more slowly, require much more repetition, and ultimately plateau at a lower level. The rehabilitation methodology we present is intended for individuals who were born with at least borderline normal range intelligence.

By using a fourth grade reading level as a cutoff, individuals with severe dyslexia and the mentally retarded are screened out. It is quite possible that someone with a fourth grade reading level has learning disabilities, but they would have reached a level to allow them to benefit from the program. Most of the software programs that adults and adolescents would find interesting require at least a fourth grade reading level. Although reading deficits are a serious problem that hampers daily functioning, NEAR is not a solution for illiteracy. Special education teachers, and specific reading remediation software and instructional materials are more appropriate for an adolescent or adult who can barely read or is unable to read.

The selection criteria dealing with time since drug or alcohol detox and whether or not someone is actively using these substances are intended to avoid potentially unproductive expenditure of clinical resources. Individuals who are actively undergoing detoxification from drugs or alcohol are not physically in a state to start focusing on cognitive skills. Furthermore, the impairments that they show immediately after detox typically improve spontaneously to some degree over a period of 3–6 weeks. For example, they may show attentional problems that would spontaneously remit within 4 weeks after detox. Therefore, it is difficult to know exactly what to target until their condition stabilizes. The cognitive treatment may be applied in detox settings to expedite cognitive recovery, but it also is reasonable to wait until it is clear what the more enduring cognitive problems are. Providing cognitive rehabilitation to someone who is actively using is likely to have little benefit because one cannot adequately assess what the enduring deficits are. That does not mean that the substance abuser who has rare and occasional relapses should be barred from the program. Relapses are common in the psychiatric population, and they can be handled by restructuring the sessions or taking a break until some stabilization occurs.

People with mental illness can also have neurologic conditions that cause cognitive impairment. Some people have had head injury; others have central nervous system diseases like multiple sclerosis or lupus. The approach to cognitive deficits in neurologic patients is and should be different than that taken with psychiatric patients. Their deficits, their experiences with learning, and the course of their illness can be quite different. Many of the cognitive remediation programs for people with head injury are not equipped to deal with the problems that arise when treating someone with persistent mental illness. However, given the expertise of these programs, if the head-injured psychiatric patient is reasonably stable from a psychiatric standpoint, they stand much to gain from attending the cognitive remediation programs for people with head injury. However, this benefit is likely to dwindle over time, as the person stabilizes and adjusts to his disability. At that point they may benefit from a program that is more oriented to treating the cognitive deficits associated with their psychiatric disability.

Communication With the Treatment Team

Once the treatment is underway, feedback should be given to the referring clinician about the appropriateness of the referral, the treatment goals, and progress that is made. This can be best achieved by either attending team meetings or writing treatment update notes. Just as it is important for other clinicians working with the client to hear about the progress being made in cognitive rehabilitation, it is essential for the cognitive rehabilitation clinician to keep abreast of the progress in other treatment modalities. It is not uncommon for progress to be uneven, and it is instructive to learn the settings and approaches that work best for any given client. Only by working together can the involved clinicians and client optimize the likelihood of treatment success.

Start-up Time Frames

It typically takes several months to establish a cognitive rehabilitation program, because there is equipment to purchase, staff to train, and a referral process to implement. A typical time frame would be 2–3 months to purchase equipment and supplies, hire or designate a clinician, and set up a space; 1–2 months for initial training of the clinician; and 3 months to build up to a caseload of 15 clients. The commitment and support of administrative and senior staff, and the enthusiasm and talent of the cognitive rehabilitation clinician will expedite the process. Once the program is set up and running, it will again require several months to take hold, and communication with referring staff is essential during this period. When clients start to give positive feedback and their successes become noticeable, the merits of the program will become self-evident.

Following is a list of materials and supplies necessary for starting a cognitive remediation program with group sizes of six.

Supply List

<u>Furniture</u>
One locking file cabinet
Sturdy tables for the computers
Seven desk chairs
One bulletin board
One desk for the clinician

<u>Computer Hardware</u>
Six computers
Six sets of speakers
Six computer monitors (display size 15–17 inches)
Six surge protectors
Four headsets

<u>Computer Software (see Chapter 4 for more information on choosing software)</u>
Four copies Math Arena™
Three copies Where in the USA is Carmen Sandiego?®
One copy Thinkin' Things™ Collection 1
Four copies Thinkin' Things™ Collection 2
Four copies Thinkin' Things™ Collection 3
Two copies Zoombinis Mountain Rescue™
Two copies Zoombinis Logical Journey™
One copy Hot Dog Stand
Two copies Math for the Real World™
Two copies Grammar for the Real World™
One copy Cross Country USA
Two copies The Factory
One copy How the West was One + Three × Four
One copy Frogger
One copy Puzzle Tanks™

Referrals typically come from other clinicians or family members. If the clinician at The Learning Center, sees clients in another capacity, say as a case manager or therapist, he is in an excellent position to identify suitable candidates for cognitive remediation. When another clinician refers a client, the steps of the referral process are as follows:

1. A clinician makes some assessment that cognitive deficits are interfering with the rehabilitation process. Urge clinicians to talk to you at this stage, so that you can help them decide if participation in the cognitive remediation program is appropriate.

2. The client's motivation and readiness to work on these problems is assessed. The clinician presents the option of attending The Learning Center.

3. The clinician completes a referral form (see appendix for a sample form).

4. If possible, the CRS reviews the client's medical record before scheduling the intake to see if there are any glaring contraindications for program entry.

5. The CRS arranges for an intake with the client.

6. If available, a brief formal psychometric assessment of cognitive functions can be made. This is an optional but highly advisable step that can provide useful information for treatment planning and outcomes monitoring.

7. After the intake, the CRS gives feedback to the clinician and client about the appropriateness of the referral and the treatment goals.

It is a good idea to arrange referrals alphabetically in a file. As each referral is processed, create a file for the client and place it in the locking file cabinet. This file will contain all information about the client's activities in the program. When a person is referred, make sure that he meets the entry requirements of the program before setting up an intake appointment. If there is important information missing that could influence a decision about acceptance, ask the clinician to supply that before scheduling the intake.

Frequently Asked Questions About the Referral Process

1. *What should I do if there are no referrals?*

    This often happens with a new program because people do not yet know how to use it. Perhaps clinicians are not aware about the program, or do not really understand how it might help their clients, or find the referral process confusing or unwieldy. To correct this situation, attend staff meetings, listen to discussion about the clients and, where appropriate, suggest that a certain individual might benefit from attending The Learning Center. Offer to fill out the referral form with the clinician. Schedule an open house and invite people into The Learning Center to show them some of the exercises you do with clients to improve problem solving skills. Post a flyer inviting clients to visit The Learning Center (see Figure 3.2 for an example).

    People will only be referred to the program if their treating clinicians are aware of the availability of the service and the ways it can help their clients. Therefore, referring clinicians should be offered education about cognitive deficits in psychiatric disorders, the ways these deficits impact in daily life, and the treatments available for cognitive dysfunction. This can be done by giving an in-service or talk, which should include some detailed explanation about the way the cognitive remediation program works, and who should be referred to it. When the discussion with the clinicians is highly interactive, it is more likely that they will develop a good understanding of the program. Use case examples, so that it becomes very clear who should be referred. This type of discussion may need to take place several times, because it takes time and experience to learn about a new treatment modality. There are other ways to make people aware of the new service. Leave the door to the room open whenever possible, invite people to try out some of the exercises, or print up a newsletter.

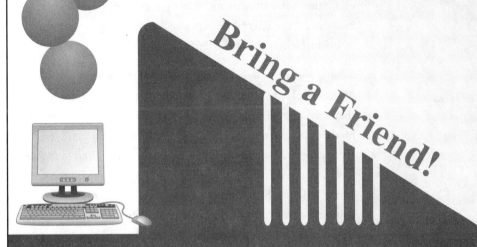

YOU ARE INVITED

TO THE OPEN HOUSE FOR THE LEARNING CENTER

Bring a Friend!

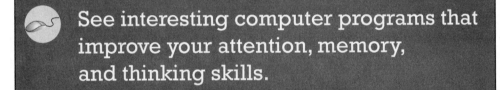

See interesting computer programs that improve your attention, memory, and thinking skills.

Find out that learning can be fun.

When: March 3rd 2–4 p.m.

Where: 6th Floor, Room 23

Figure 3.2

Sample invitation flyer.

2. *What should I do if there are too many referrals?*

Stay calm! You will get to them all in time. When a program is first starting, referrals tend to come in fits and starts. Promptly call all appropriate referrals to set up an appointment. If you delay in responding to referrals, people will not experience the program as responsive. Not all referrals work out because of scheduling problems or other events that may come up. Sometimes a person may be interested in joining the program but may be in the midst of another commitment and able to start only at a later date. However, if the referral process was a positive experience, the individual will reconnect later.

3. *What if the person does not show up for their intake?*

Many people are referred to The Learning Center precisely because they forget appointments, so it should not be surprising that some intake appointments will be missed. Call the person and say, *"I understood that you were going to come to The Learning Center on such and such a date. Did something come up?"* If the person forgot, set up a plan to help him remember the next scheduled appointment. Offer to call him the day before or the morning of the appointment. Ask the client to write down the appointment and put the information by his front door. If the person changed his mind about coming, offer to give a tour of the facility and show him the program so he can have a better idea of what it is all about. Let the referring clinician know that the person may need some extra support and encouragement to attend. Ultimately, it is essential to try to figure out why the person did not show up for the appointment and address the underlying issue with supportive, nonjudgmental interventions.

4. *How do I handle self-referrals?*

When clients self-refer, that is a sign that the program has "taken hold," that it has become a group that people want to belong to. Sometimes clients will self-refer because they have walked by and the open door has allowed them to catch a glimpse of something that seems interesting. Other times clients will hear about the program from others. The best advertisement for the program is always from the people attending it. It is not uncommon that clients attending the program will encourage their friends to join.

When someone shows interest in the program, offer to set up an intake appointment and indicate that you will speak to the other clinicians who work with the client. It is important for the client to know that you work collaboratively with the other staff.

5. *How many referrals do I need to start a group?*
    The beginning CRS should start the group with the first two referrals and then add another client every month until there are six to eight participants in the group. Starting slowly will allow the CRS to get comfortable with the procedures, and the rolling admissions usually facilitates the referral process and integration with the overall rehabilitation program. Rolling admissions to multiple groups allows the CRS to carefully consider group dynamics and best fit between a new participant and the "regulars."

Chapter 4 *Selecting Appropriate Software*

Software Selection

Building a software library is key to making the cognitive rehabilitation program a success. Having a range of software that targets different skills and offers a variety of opportunities for contextualization and personalization ensures that the program can meet the needs of a diverse population. To build a software library, the clinician must choose amongst the vast array of software available on the market. Therefore, it is important to learn how to analyze the software in order to be prepared to make informed decisions when ordering supplies. Consider the 5 Cs (cognitive, client, computer, context, and choice) when choosing software (see Table 4.1).

This checklist allows the cognitive rehabilitation specialist (CRS) to consider specific and nonspecific treatment factors when ordering software. Specific factors of treatment refer to the specific cognitive deficits that will be targeted. One of the 5 Cs, "cognitive," concerns these specific factors. The various cognitive deficits that can be targeted by educational software are discussed in the sections that follow. Ultimately, the cognitively enhancing potential of the software must be sufficiently evident to justify a client spending time on it. Nonspecific factors refer to those aspects of the software that facilitate learning without targeting a specific cognitive deficit. Three of the 5 Cs relate to nonspecific factors: "computer," "context," and "choice." Specific factors related to the client include such variables as the client's level of cognitive functioning and suitability of the content of the software. Fantasy contexts that involve morbid or violent themes are to be avoided. Clients may be required to have a minimal reading level for some software, or the task may require a prerequisite amount of

Table 4.1 Choosing Software for Cognitive Rehabilitation: A Checklist of the 5 Cs

1. COGNITIVE
   What are the target deficits to be addressed? (e.g., visual or auditory attention, verbal working memory, deductive reasoning, linear sequencing, organization, etc.)

2. CLIENT
   What are the interests and level of functioning of the individual and the context of the setting? (e.g., reading level, affective and motivational needs, suitable task content, relevance to treatment goals, etc.)

3. COMPUTER
   What are the requirements and compatibility of the software and hardware? (e.g., RAM, MAC vs. PC, operating system, hard disk vs. CD-ROM, user-friendly directions, etc.)

4. CONTEXT
   Does the software use the motivationally enhancing instructional technique of contextualizing the learning activity? Is the activity contextualized as a real-world activity or a fantasy? If it is a fantasy, is the content appropriate (e.g., no violence, not morbid), and is the story line sufficiently simple that someone with limited working memory can retain it?

5. CHOICE
   Does the software use the motivationally enhancing instructional technique of providing learner choices? Are there opportunities for the learner to choose options to adapt the activity? (e.g., multimedia format, printed output, difficulty level, automatically paced vs. specific menus, speed, etc.)

domain-specific knowledge. The client's particular interests should be reflected in the choice of software. There is a diversity of content ranging from pioneer adventures, detective work, and truck driving to trading stock and word games, which should facilitate personalization of the learning experience. Further discussion of prerequisite client skills is presented later on. Motivationally enhancing features of software selections, such as contextualization and choice, should be assessed as well. Flexibility and a wide range of difficulty are necessary prerequisites when improvement and competency are treatment goals. Further discussion of adaptability of software will be illustrated with examples of software analysis later in the chapter.

Practical aspects of compatibility with the available computer hardware must be elicited. Some of the available software require a CD-ROM drive, although many can be installed and opened from the hard drive. In order to accommodate software, especially the new multimedia software, consideration of the hardware is essential. Most CD-ROM software is hybrid and runs equally well on PCs or Macs; however, not all software runs on the Microsoft® Vista platform. Minimum central processing unit (CPU) requirements include hard disk space for 20 programs, adequate RAM (random access memory) and processing speed, and speakers with compatible sound drivers. Optional headphones, accommodation for Internet access, and a color printer are attractive peripherals.

Most of the software used in the Neuropsychological and Educational Approach to Cognitive Remediation (NEAR) is available through educational resources, although we also use web-based activities (e.g., www.gamesforthebrain.com; www.happy-neuron.com) and some software created specifically for treating cognition in psychiatric populations. Table 4.2 offers a list of some Web sites that provide information and sales of relevant software, but the reader is advised to periodically do web searches, because new software companies are always entering the market, especially now that there is so much interest in treating cognition in the aging.

These publishers are reliable sources for technical assistance and provide ongoing support when needed. They are constantly developing new product lines and upgrades of various software programs, some of which build on familiar procedures, characters, and content, and many of which follow a developmental sequence. Other modifications to existing software take into account the ongoing improvement in computer technology.

Many of the suppliers have arrangements for preview of materials for up to 30 days and guarantee refunds or exchanges. Catalogs are updated, and promotional sale items are advertised and include preview disks

Table 4.2 Online Software Resources

www.knowledgeadventure.com
www.sunburst.com
www.ccvsoftware.com
www.edmark.com
www.learningcompany.com
www.positscience.com

and free software. Supplementary materials such as teacher manuals and handouts may be included, which may be useful for noncomputer activities or small group projects.

Software orders are initially based on the descriptions provided in the catalog. Because educational publishers are in the market of developing software suitable for classroom settings, they use language suitable for making learning objectives explicit. They provide information pertinent to the actual content and process of approaching the materials covered in any given software program so that one has an understanding of what to expect when the software arrives.

Many of the software descriptions emphasize the age level, applicability to educational curriculum, and the content vis-à-vis subject matter (i.e., history, geography, science, mathematics). As the software will be used for a different purpose than it is marketed for, the CRS needs to learn how to evaluate software for applicability to cognitive remediation. For example, a program marketed to teach mathematics might prove to be excellent at remediating problem solving skills and a program marketed to grades 5-8 may be excellent for people with cognitive dysfunction.

Once the software is ordered, a thorough review of the activity is necessary in order to maximize the utility of each particular selection in the software library. Because the focus is not on the educational content but, rather, the viability of the program as a tool for cognitive remediation, a thorough familiarity with procedures and processes related to running the program successfully is imperative. An example of a sample computer task analysis is provided in Figure 4.1. A blank analysis form for your use is provided in the appendix.

This generic outline can be used as a guide when the CRS approaches the software task for the first time. Copies of each computer task analysis can be kept with the software packaging.

This thorough description and analysis facilitates awareness of all the aspects of the program for appropriate treatment planning. By gaining experience and extensive practice in the analysis of the software, the CRS can generate a more streamlined listing using simple analyses, as noted in Table 4.3, which may suffice for quick reference.

Name of Software Program:	Fripple House (Thinkin' Things™ Collection 3 by Edmark)
Description of Activity:	The goal is to place the correct "fripple" into the designated living quarters according to the written instructions.
Reading Level Required:	Minimum 2nd grade reading level

Other Prerequisite Skills Needed:

(1) Color vision and discrimination (2) Click and drag technique with the mouse

Cognitive Deficits That Can Be Addressed:

(1) Verbal working memory (2) Deductive reasoning (3) Initiation and sustained effort for goal-directed actions (4) Categorization and classification of objects (5) Organizational strategies (6) Ability to use feedback to monitor and revise strategies

Goal Properties

Clearly defined goal is to place the fripples in the correct apartment.

As levels advance, more steps are needed to reach the goal.

Adaptability of Task:

Continuum of difficulty is available, starting with concrete and explicit verbal descriptions to implicit and abstract verbal operations.

Level of difficulty adjusts according to accuracy and individual performance.

Allows for self-pacing.

Hints are available to aid progress.

Multimedia Experience:

Colorful images, encouraging feedback ("you're a great detective!"), and visually stimulating scenes.

Mediation by Therapist:

Opportunities to foster visual scanning, self-monitoring, and learning strategies. Task demands can be increased by manipulating level of difficulty manually.

Overall Strengths and Weaknesses:

Untimed, interesting, reinforcing, cognitively challenging activity.

May need to be sensitive to client's interpretations of "fripples" as childish.

Figure 4.1

An example of a generic computer task analysis.

Table 4.3 Samples of Computer Software for Cognitive Rehabilitation

Name of program	Task analysis at a glance
1. Where in the USA/World is Carmen Sandiego?®	Used to improve problem solving, organization, working memory, reasoning, sustained effort, verbal memory, planning, dual tasking.
2. Oregon Trail	Ability to work on tasks with distal goals, learning multiple steps, planning and organization, memory, attention to detail, sustained effort, decision making.
3. Thinkin' Things™ Collection 3 (Stocktopus, Fripple House)	Deductive reasoning, categorization of information in order to solve problems, working memory, sequencing and planning.
4. Puzzle Tanks™	Problem solving, mental flexibility, comparison, synthesis, mathematical deductions.
5. Word Attack 3 (Hat Attack aka Slime Game)	Verbal memory, divided attention, sustained effort, visual scanning and reaction time, information processing speed.
6. The Factory	Nonverbal reasoning, spatial orientation, visual memory, visual discrimination, sequencing, planning, working memory.
7. Carmen Word Detective	Problem solving, sequential reasoning, initiation of action, planning ahead, strategic thinking, mental flexibility, working memory.
8. Spell It® Deluxe (Leap to Complete)	Vigilance, reaction time, auditory processing, verbal working memory, processing speed, visual scanning.
9. How the West Was $1 + 3 \times 4$	Use of mathematical problem solving, decision making, organization and planning steps and sequences in order to reach a desired solution, attention.
10. Venn (Math Arena™)	Problem solving, processing speed, categorization, deductive reasoning, working memory.

Quick reference listings are also helpful when managing a large software library and client caseload. Whereas this simpler analysis keeps an organized listing of target deficits, an extended analysis increases the clinician's familiarity with the nuances of each particular activity. For example, eye–hand coordination and reaction time might be important prerequisite skills needed for one software activity, whereas sustained attention for tasks with distal goals might be an important element of another. Therefore, it is recommended that the generic outline be used by staff for extensive analysis and maximal familiarity.

Use of guidelines for software analysis is imperative when training new staff to implement cognitive remediation. Although experienced clinicians may automatically and implicitly analyze the activities that fit with the client's interests, abilities, and cognitive needs, the new CRS will find this a challenging task. The step-by-step analysis introduces the concepts to treatment providers who are sorting out information on a variety of levels and are just developing the necessary skills for working in The Learning Center. Further analyses using an outline specific to the NEAR model are described in the sections that follow.

Targeted Deficits

Although selecting the appropriate software depends on the salient characteristics of the individual being treated and the context of treatment, the primary focus is to determine the cognitive deficits that can be addressed within each particular software program. For example, opportunities for auditory versus visual attention, sustained concentration, visual scanning, verbal versus visual memory, sequencing and organization, initiation, goal setting, maintenance of set, and problem solving, among other targeted areas, must be delineated.

As the major areas of cognitive impairment targeted for treatment involve processes related to attention, memory, processing speed, and problem solving, software programs should be analyzed for opportunities to address these needs. When exploring software, look for these opportunities by investigating the procedures and reflecting on the cognitive processes that are engaged during the task. Although each cognitive process is separately analyzed, one must remember that multiple demands are being placed on the individual for information processing while working on computer software. These are not always sequential or isolated, but frequently overlapping demands that recapitulate the natural course of events. In fact, it is this aspect of simulation that is capitalized on in the NEAR model, rather than using software that engage drill and practice of an isolated cognitive function. Therefore, using the questions provided, the following areas of cognition should be noted when analyzing software activities.

Attention

What type of attention is required—selective, divided, or simultaneous? Does one have to scan stimuli and choose a particular feature? Or does one have to alternately observe different features? What are the opportunities for simultaneous processing of information? Are there subtle or obvious features that must be attended to in order to succeed in the software? Can changes be made to the demands on attention, such as increasing the number of stimuli, limiting the time, and eliminating extraneous information? What level of distraction is tolerated while still successfully completing the task?

Concentration

What are the opportunities for building concentration and sustained attention? How does the interaction between the user and software demands engage one's endurance? What are the pleasurable aspects of successfully attending over time?

Memory

What are requirements for immediate recall of information? How is information presented—using auditory cues, pictorial cues, symbol representation, or written expression? Is information presented in various forms simultaneously and redundantly? Can information be repeated? Are there opportunities to store and retrieve information (e.g., use of a journal or Post-it® notes) as a mnemonic memory aid? Are the demands related to working memory versus short-term memory? Is it difficult to learn the procedures for running the software? How can procedural memory (e.g., memory for the procedures to operate the software) be enhanced with cues that are available? Are the demands for verbal memory or visual memory dominant? How can mnemonic strategies be integrated into the task?

Basic Reasoning Skills

What level of abstraction is required to interpret information? How can information be compared and contrasted? Is there a readily apparent principle that guides analysis in a deductive process? Does gathering data build concepts in an inductive manner? What are the software tools that support reasoning skills when an individual cannot sufficiently draw conclusions on her own?

Simple Problem Solving

Is the problem/goal identifiable and manageable? Are the steps for successful completion to answering the puzzle or problem sequential and organized? Is there ample time given to complete the tasks or to break the task down into manageable parts? Is the content of the problem interesting and stimulating to sustain interest? What types of strategies can be used during the problem solving process? Does the software include good instructions or help menus for self-exploration?

Complex Problem Solving

In addition to queries regarding simple problem solving software, what aspects of the software can be taught by observation or trial-and-error learning? Is experimentation allowed? Are there opportunities for summaries and integration of material (e.g., use of journal)? Can the steps required to reach the goal be readily identified and remembered?

Prerequisite Client Skills

Computers can be intimidating as well as inspiring because of their high status and high-profile image in contemporary culture. They can also be challenging for clients who have difficulties with perceptual mechanisms, motor control, visual pursuit and scanning, and educational deficits, such as poor reading skills, or cognitive rigidity or inflexibility. Therefore, in addition to cognitive functioning, there are many aspects of client skills that must be considered when using computers.

When software is evaluated, the demands on information processing using particular perceptual, visual, and motor cues are quite important. Matching software to the skill level of the client is an art so that client frustration about her lack of prerequisite skills does not impede remediation of cognition.

Important prerequisite skills to consider include *perceptual factors* such as left–right discrimination and figure-ground processing; *visual factors* such as visual acuity and smooth eye pursuit for visual scanning; and *motor factors* such as eye–hand coordination, reaction time, and speed of motor processing, and praxis or motor planning skills. Many clients using medication have abnormal movements such as tremors, tardive dyskinesia, or myoclonic jerks that interfere with good mouse control. As substituting the keyboard for mouse manipulation is not always possible, trying wrist weights may assist some clients with better motor control because of the increased kinesthetic and proprioceptive feedback. The computer's mouse settings can also be altered so that the mouse is more or less sensitive and responsive to the user's hand movements. Other helpful features of the software include modification of speed of characters for those who are processing information slowly. A technique to enhance appropriate visual scanning and eye–hand coordination include exercises devoted to exploring every inch of the computer screen using a "window-washing" motion, up and down, systematically covering the screen. Many software activities also promote this movement in a goal-directed manner and can be useful in enhancing these required skills.

Goal Properties

It is important to consider whether the goal properties of the task are appropriate for the client because activities with distal or poorly defined goals would be difficult for someone with working memory and reasoning deficits. Consider if the goal is well-defined, for example, to sort items according to a given principle or if the goal can be satisfied in multiple ways, for example, to make money running a simulated hot dog stand. The proximity of the goal is also an important consideration because people with poor attention and low self-esteem will need immediate feedback and short exercises. An activity like Combo Cubes from Math Arena™ can be accomplished in a minute, whereas Grammar for the Real World™ can take hours.

Promotion of Intrinsic Motivation and Task Engagement

The NEAR model focuses on educational principles and learning theory. In order to effectively apply the principles of the model, one must accept some basic tenets proposed by Lieber & Semmel (1985) for use when teaching "disabled" clients. We suggest that effective teaching tools and activities must include the following features for the clients:

1) Intrinsically motivating

2) Active use of information

3) Multisensory strategies

4) Frequent feedback

5) Control over learning process

6) Positive reinforcement

7) Application of newly acquired skill in contextualized formats

8) Challenging but not frustrating (e.g., errorless learning)

A key component is the idea that intrinsic motivation, defined as valuing or enjoyment of task activities, is an essential ingredient for the learning process. Intrinsic motivation can be increased or decreased by many events (Dweck, 1985):

1. It is *increased* by choice, emphasis on a strategy approach, specific and persuasive feedback, and feeling competent in the face of challenge, that is, information events for *self-determination.*

2. It is increased when *learning goals are emphasized.*

3. It is *decreased* by external rewards or pressures such as awards, deadlines, and surveillance, that is, controlling events. These aspects *emphasize performance goals.*

Therefore, in order to promote intrinsic motivation and task involvement during learning activities that use computer software, one must look for the features that allow the learner to optimize self-determination and decrease performance goals in favor of learning goals. This enhances self-evaluation, which is an important aspect of guiding one's own learning experience.

As these principles have been applied to educational software (Bitter, Camuse, & Durbin, 1993; Hannafin & Peck, 1988), they relate to the nonspecific treatment factors that facilitate learning without targeting any one specific cognitive activity. They are pervasive factors that affect the entire treatment experience. They include the following characteristics:

1. Contextualization of the learning in either a fantasy or real-life simulation

2. Choices that increase motivation and learning, such as choosing difficulty level, pacing, competition versus cooperation, and adjusting sound features

3. Personalization so that the learner enters into the activity of interest as an identifiable agent

4. The opportunity to make mistakes without experiencing failure, the opportunity to try out solutions and learn from mistakes

The process of learning is enhanced when contextualization, personalization, and choice are experienced during the educational activity because of their positive effects on increasing intrinsic motivation (Cordova & Lepper, 1996). Therefore, it is of paramount importance to consider all of the nonspecific factors, in addition to the specific targeted cognitive deficits, when selecting and analyzing software. See the form in the appendix for an example of an outline to follow when evaluating software in accordance with what is known about educational benefits. You may photocopy the form from this book or use it as a model for creating your own. Examples of how this outline has been applied to various software selections are shown in Figures 4.2 through 4.5.

Software Program Name/Manufacturer:

Spell It® Deluxe by Davidson®

Activity:

Leap to Complete

1. Cognitive deficits targeted by the software:

Vigilance

Reaction time

Processing speed

Verbal working memory

Simultaneous processing of two information inputs

Visual scanning

2. Required knowledge base:

Domain specific knowledge: Spelling; language arts

Reading level: Range from 1st grade to college level

3. Working memory/Attention requirements:

Emphasizes selective and sustained and divided attention, and uses verbal working memory (i.e., hear the word, remember it long enough to know the letters that are missing to start the search)

Figure 4.2

Example of software analysis using education principles 1–3.

Software Program Name/Manufacturer:

Word Attack® by Davidson®

Activity:

Maze

4. Motivation:

Intrinsic:

Sense of personal causation is high

Appeal of progress and achievement

Recognizing strengths in crystallized intelligence

Curiosity about the journey

Figure 4.3

Example of software analysis using educational principles 4–6.

Extrinsic:

Points scored

Beating the clock

Eating the goodies

Zapping the bugs

(These give input about competence, which can increase intrinsic motivation)

5. Depth of Engagement:

Divided attention requires active and good depth of processing for recall

Recall of previous definitions viewed

Planning the course in maze

Multitasking; integrative actions

6. Opportunities for self-perceived competence:

Feedback provided: Eats words and gets points

Experience of success: Multiple levels; repeatable; mastery of coordinated efforts (motor actions)

Figure 4.3 *continued*

Software Program Name/Manufacturer:

Thinkin' Things™ Collection 3 by Edmark

Activity:

Fripple House

7. Multisensory Presentation:

Level of stimulation:

Colorful

Encouraging feedback ("great detective")

Visually stimulating

Engaging characters

Figure 4.4

Example of software analysis using educational principles 7–9.

8. Contextualization:

Fantasy or real-life simulation:

Contextualized as tenants in an apartment house, but the tenants are fantasy creatures

Single, multiple contexts:

Single context of an apartment house, but multiple houses shown

Relevance to daily life:

Use of sorting, categorization, attributes, planning ahead (e.g., laundry, budgeting)

9. Learner Controls/Choice

Difficulty levels:

Graded; changing with accuracy

Competitive versus Cooperative:

Ability to get hints; willingness to keep trying

Other:

Self-evaluation and monitoring for accuracy

Figure 4.4 *continued*

Software Program Name/Manufacturer:

Where in the World is Carmen Sandiego?® by Broderbund®

10. Opportunities for practice

With different cues/context:

New cities; new people; new cases; same procedure

Within/between difficulty levels:

Variability of clues; looking for congruence; ability to do research on database; increased difficulty with progress and cases won.

11. Personalization:

Sign-in; keeping track of cases; promotions; competing with peers ("how did so-and-so do?"); attention and comments from chief; newspaper banner announcing outcome; familiarity and prior exposure to TV show

Figure 4.5

Example of software analysis using educational principles 10–11.

Involving clients in the selection and evaluation of software is an effective way of engaging them as active members of The Learning Center, whose opinions matter. This enhances self-esteem while promoting analytic thinking, metacognition, and verbal communication. Many software suppliers include evaluation forms that can be distributed to clients for their feedback. Clients can also fill out a reaction questionnaire after a treatment session to reflect on their enjoyment and the pertinent skills that were addressed by the particular program. In addition, clients can write about their experiences with software activities so that other program participants can read what their peers think about individual programs. These reviews can be included in a newsletter published by The Learning Center. Examples of client reviews are included in Figure 4.6.

In addition to communication with peers, the written expression allows clients to organize their thinking processes and integrate their perceptions of what therapeutic benefit they receive from the activity. This facilitates self-awareness and self-evaluation, both valuable skills that can enhance metacognition.

> "Everyone in the Learning Center is different; therefore, everyone will not like the same things. However, I like the software program The Factory. This particular program is challenging. You must plan ahead in order to make the product that they ask for. Each machine that the product goes through does something different to the product. One machine will turn the product; another machine will punch holes in the product. There are three levels of difficulty: easy, medium, and hard. In order to make the product, you must determine what machines and in what order they should be in to make the desired item. In addition to planning ahead, the following thinking skills are developed: paying attention to details, following directions, experimenting, taking risks, using your imagination by picturing the outcome, applying information in one situation after another, reasoning by comparison and contrast.........AND YOU HAVE A GOOD TIME DOING IT!"

Figure 4.6

Examples of client reviews of software programs.

"Fripple House helps you to concentrate on detail, organization, and decision making. It is stimulating and challenging, especially when you are learning it for the first time. (It looks easier than it is.) The instructions can be understood. There are different degrees of difficulty, which requires more attention to detail. The colorful icons make this program very interesting to look at."

"The Hot Dog Stand was a very challenging game for me. I had to use my memory to pay attention to a lot of details when preparing for an event. Some of the tasks involved determining the number of people expected at an event, which was based upon the weather, time, and type of event. This information can be obtained by looking through the book "How to Run with the Big Dogs." After reading this book, I was ready to order food to sell at the stand. I compared the prices for food at the different suppliers and purchased from the most reliable. One thing to remember is not to over order hot dogs or buns because they will spoil. I will continue to use Hot Dog Stand to improve my reasoning and memory."

"Today in the lab I worked on Cross Country USA for the first time. It was a real challenge learning how to play the game. I learned about budgeting money, and I learned about what truck drivers actually have to go through when they are hauling their merchandise. I studied the map and directions in which I had to go, then I chose really carefully either "north, south, east, or west and points in between" on the compass. I am happy to say I reached my destination and I acquired all my commodities. I started in San Francisco, CA, then I went to Los Angeles, and then I went to Tucson, AZ, and then onto Albuquerque, NM. To summarize, this program helped me to think logically in new situations, plan ahead, and focus on the goal and pay attention to details along the way. I got a real bang from Cross Country but no flat tires!"

Figure 4.6 *continued*

In summary, the CRS must thoughtfully review each software selection in order to build the most accommodating software library for a particular setting. The CRS must analyze the software so that the specific and nonspecific factors of cognitive remediation strategies are maximized. The clients may offer their reactions in order to verify that the selections satisfy and stimulate learning opportunities for the best treatment outcomes. Table 4.4 is a listing of a sample software library with programs that incorporate the principles reviewed in this chapter. This listing is

Table 4.4 Sample Inventory of Learning Center Supplies

Software Selection

Math Arena™
Grammar for the Real World™
Math for the Real World™
Cross Country USA
Zoombinis Mountain Rescue™
Zoombinis Logical Journey™
Oregon Trail
The Factory
Hot Dog Stand: The Works
How the West Was $1 + 3 \times 4$
Puzzle Tanks™
Thinkin' Things™ Collection 1
Thinkin' Things™ Collection 2
Thinkin' Things™ Collection 3
Where in the U.S.A. is Carmen Sandiego?®
Where in the World is Carmen Sandiego?®
Carmen Sandiego Think Quick Challenge®
Ultimate Word Attack 3
Spell It® Deluxe
Super Solvers Mission Think
More Brain Games (sold at www.onhandsoftware.com)
Web-based activities:
www.Gamesforthebrain.com
www.happy-neuron.com

not definitive because educational software is updated and new programs are developed at a rapid pace. However, it represents a selection of software titles derived by following the principles of analysis described in this chapter and illustrate the extent of diversity in available software titles that supports the NEAR model of treatment.

Chapter 5   *Intake and Assessment*

The intake appointment is the first sustained contact the person has with The Learning Center, and it is important that this be a positive experience. The person should be made to feel welcome and comfortable. Many people will experience great trepidation because they have had repeated experiences of failure in learning settings. They expect that this will be yet one more negative experience. For many, it is an act of great courage to come to the intake. They are in essence saying, "Even though I have failed in the past, I WILL TRY AGAIN." The cognitive rehabilitation specialist (CRS) must convey respect for their willingness to try to learn, and appreciation for their anxiety. A calm and accepting manner is usually experienced positively. The very fact that the person is there is a testament to one of the most positive aspects of human potential—the desire to learn. That must be fostered and encouraged.

Primary Goals of Intake

1. To provide a positive experience for the client

2. To engage the client in the program

3. To gather sufficient information about learning style, cognitive problems, areas of personal interest, and ability level so that an initial treatment plan can be formulated

4. To set up a schedule and session plan

Meeting With the Client

After introductions, ask the client how he heard about the program and what about it he found interesting. Ask how he thinks it might help him.

The person may not be sure; after all he may not know much about the program, and may not have a great awareness of his areas of impairment. Tell the client about The Learning Center. Explain that it is a place where people can improve their learning skills and find enjoyment in learning. Explain that the program utilizes computers and inquire about the client's level of computer experience. Explain that some of the skills addressed in the program include paying attention, remembering, and solving problems. Ask the person if he wants to work on any specific areas. Ask if he finds that his attention wanders when people talk to him. This discussion should allow you to assess awareness of deficit. Notice also that people have different levels of comfort in discussing problems. Learn the language each person uses to describe his problems, and stick with that initially. Later you can introduce new terms.

The information we suggest you gather together with the client is outlined in the Assessment and Treatment Plan form provided in the appendix. This is a form that the client can also look at. You may photocopy it from the book and distribute to your clients if applicable. The questions serve to guide you to the general areas that you should ask the client about: school, work, learning experiences, identified cognitive difficulties, and goals. Within each area there are many questions you could ask.

School

- Aside from the highest grade obtained, did you repeat or skip any grades?

- Were you in special education, or ever diagnosed with learning disabilities or attention-deficit hyperactivity disorder?

- What did/does/would interest you at school?

- What were the subjects you did best in?

- Was school a positive experience?

- How did your family view school? Was an education valued?

Work

■ What kind of work have you done?

■ What kind of work do you want to be doing?

■ What is the longest period you worked in the same job?

Learning Style

The main point of discussing learning style is to start the process of self-awareness about the client's approach to learning. In fact, most people learn through multiple modalities. Nevertheless, by asking the client if he is a "morning person" or a better listener than reader, you help the client to think of himself as having a learning style and start him thinking about his strengths and weaknesses.

Treatment Goals

It is important to meld the goals of cognitive remediation with the overall treatment goals. The client should see this from the start.

■ What goals have you set for yourself?

■ What goals are you working on in treatment?

■ How do cognitive deficits interfere with attainment of these goals?

Formal and Informal Assessments

The initial assessment is intended to give enough information to determine if the person is suitable for cognitive remediation and to provide clues about how to best engage him in learning. NEAR uses a naturalistic, fluid assessment process, whereby behaviors and reactions are analyzed over time to point to potential treatment strategies. Nonetheless, it is valuable to have an understanding of the client's basic strengths and weaknesses in order to have a starting point to begin working with the client. This is ideally ascertained through a combination of formal and informal assessments.

Formal assessments can be extremely useful because they allow for a more fine-tuned approach to treatment planning and give a baseline measure against which to compare posttreatment outcome. The choice of tests will depend largely upon the staffing of the program, because many tests require specialized training to administer. It is problematic to have the CRS do formal testing as the role of a tester conflicts with that of a clinician, and it is important that the client mainly sees the CRS as someone who facilitates a learning process. We have had success using computerized assessments because clients find them interesting to do, and the CRS can again be a facilitator—here facilitating the taking of the test. Computerized tests also have the advantage of being easy to administer, and many have data management capabilities. We have not found that extended neuropsychological test batteries are a necessary prerequisite for doing cognitive remediation; rather, targeted assessment of relevant outcome skills is preferable.

Formal assessment can be done in two ways: (1) psychometric measures administered by a psychologist and (2) computer-administered software or web-based assessment packages. It is important to recognize that any formal assessment can be experienced as threatening and anxiety provoking. If there is some concern that this will be the case for a given client, formal assessment can be postponed until the third session, at which point the person is hopefully sufficiently engaged to view the testing as a way of marking progress.

Informal assessment can combine brief measures, interviews, self-report questionnaires, and team feedback. One aspect of the informal assessment is a brief test of reading to ascertain grade level. Reading level is important to gauge because it correlates highly with intellectual level, can give a clue as to the presence of learning disabilities and problems acquiring knowledge, and indicates the appropriate software. Many software programs require a minimum fourth grade reading level. There are many tests of reading to choose from; we have most often used the Wide Range Achievement Test—Reading subtest (WRAT). Although this test assesses single word reading, it does not evaluate passage comprehension. Formal tests of passage comprehension exist, or the CRS can ask the client to read a brief paragraph from an interesting magazine or newspaper and check for comprehension by asking questions about the content.

Attention and concentration are informally assessed by measuring the person's ability to stay on task. Does the person need to get up after a few minutes? Is he able to attend to questions, to sit and do the problem solving screening, and sit through an initial computer software demonstration? Is he easily distracted by features of the room or noises?

Self-esteem can be assessed not only for the obvious reason but to give another chance to look at reading ability, attention, self-awareness, and coping style. The Rosenberg Self-Esteem Scale is available on the web and allows the person to score it himself. This immediately draws the client into an active role, where he is self-evaluating.

A problem solving exercise is given to provide some assessment of critical thinking. The level of difficulty can vary; it can be useful to have a few exercises readily available and pick the one that seems most appropriate. We typically give a fourth grade level task because many clients find that difficult, and it is in any case better to choose a task that will not be overwhelming (see page 66 for an example). Look to see how the person approaches the task. Does he have an organized approach? Does the person lose his purpose halfway through the exercise? Does the person get irritated and impatient, or persist and self-correct?

A client's observation of his own perceived deficits can be useful information as well, and should be included in the informal assessment. This information can be elicited during the interview, or the client can complete a short self-report questionnaire (see page 67 for an example).

You may photocopy both the problem solving exercise and the client self-report from the book and distribute to your clients.

A Problem Solving Assessment Task

How good are your problem solving skills?

Elephants live to be very old. One family of elephants has five members. Can you figure out the age of each elephant? Their names are Morris, Tamsen, Jenny, Bobby, and Sally. Their ages are 4, 8, 11, 29, and 35.

1. Bobby is older than Morris and Jenny.
2. Morris is 7 years older than Jenny.
3. Bobby was born after Sally.

	4	8	11	29	35	
						Morris
						Tamsen
						Jenny
						Bobby
						Sally

Thinking Skills Self-Appraisal

Use the following scale to rate yourself:

SCALE: 0 = Never

1 = Rarely

2 = Occasionally

3 = Frequently

4 = Most of the time

5 = Always

CIRCLE YOUR ANSWER:

1.   I have trouble concentrating.

        0   1   2   3   4   5

2.   I have trouble paying attention to conversations.

        0   1   2   3   4   5

3.   I have difficulty with my memory.

        0   1   2   3   4   5

4.   When I have things to do, I sometimes don't know where to start.

        0   1   2   3   4   5

5.   I have trouble finishing what I start.

        0   1   2   3   4   5

6.   I have difficulty figuring out and solving problems.

        0   1   2   3   4   5

Rank order the following list of problems by placing a
#1 next to the problem area that is most important for you to work on,
#2 next to the next most important problem area for you to work on,
#3 and #4 next to the problem areas with the least priority for you to work on.

_____ ATTENTION

_____ MEMORY

_____ BEING ORGANIZED

_____ FIGURING OUT PROBLEMS

Common Situations That Arise During Intake

The Person Who Is Great at Everything

This is the person who comes to the program just to "check it out." Some people will say that everything is fine, that they have excellent attention, memory, and other skills. Even though you may know this is not the case, do not confront them. Their need to say everything is perfect suggests that they are not at all comfortable discussing problems. One of the goals of treatment will be to change that, but that will only happen when the person has a sufficient bank of positive experiences and has gathered enough experiences of being genuinely competent to allow himself to reveal his flaws. For the purposes of the intake, you have learned a lot about his learning style. Instead of asking people about their problems, ask what they like to do. Put them on a task early on saying, "Would you like to try this?" After they have done something on the computer, say that you need some information about them so that you can steer them to activities they will like. Then proceed with the intake.

The Person Who Says Little and Does Not Volunteer Any Information

These quiet people may briefly answer your questions, but talking seems to make them uncomfortable. If that is the case, do not expect a long conversation, instead stay action oriented. Ask your questions, ask them to do the informal assessment tasks, and as soon as possible give them a computer exercise that you think will engage them for 10 min. Sometimes it is better to have two brief positive meetings than one long meeting that makes the client overly anxious.

The Person Who Wants Things "My Way"

These restless, energetic people stride into the room and immediately want to try all the computer exercises. They have little patience for your questions and just as little patience for learning how to use any computer program. Schedules, routines, questions, rules—all this seems unbearably constraining. They may view you with suspicion or irritation and be quick to disagree with even innocuous things that you say. It is best to keep initial meetings with these people brief, perhaps 20–30 min. A calm, firm manner will facilitate the interview, and do not hesitate to redirect them if they stray from the topic. After 15 min of gathering information, give them some time to work on a highly structured, easy to use exercise. Rather than asking what they want, give simple directives. "There is a software program you can try now." Usually, the less said the better because these people are not good listeners. From the start, it is important to provide these people with considerable structure but sufficient distance that they feel in control.

Setting Up a Schedule

At the end of the first meeting, a schedule needs to be set for 2–3 sessions a week. Help clients find hours they can reasonably be expected to attend, and emphasize the importance of arriving on time. If a client regularly carries a schedule or planner, make sure he enters the new appointments. If the client does not carry a calendar or schedule, give him a copy of his session times along with your name and office phone number in case he needs to call and cancel a session. Encourage clients to carry their schedules with them until coming to The Learning Center becomes a regular part of their routines.

Chapter 6   *Treatment Planning*

The treatment plan is intended to focus the cognitive rehabilitation specialist (CRS) and to provide a structure or template for the first few weeks of sessions. It is not a static document. Every week or two, the CRS should consider her observations of the client, the idiosyncrasies and problems that are revealed, and think about what will best help them. For the seasoned clinician this comes naturally, and the treatment plan serves mainly as a record keeper. In the first year that a CRS is working, the treatment plan is an essential document that helps refine her thinking about the cases. The treatment plan is guided by the ongoing, informal, fluid assessment of the client. To formulate the initial treatment plan, start with the steps outlined in the sections that follow.

Identify Cognitive Deficits to Target in Treatment

The informal assessments done at intake, coupled with the reports of the referring clinician and client, should guide this process. Although most clients have problems with attention, memory, and problem solving, the relative degree of these deficits and the context and ways in which they manifest will differ.

Identify Need for External Structure

It is wise to assume that the client will require more structure in the beginning of treatment, but people vary in exactly how much structure they need. If the initial assessment indicated no knowledge of working with computers, a low educational level, and considerable problems with attention, this person will likely need highly structured exercises that are not too stimulating (i.e., without multisensory effects) and have goals that are obtainable in a few obvious steps. Such clients also need considerable individualized attention initially, so that it may be best to pair them with clients who are more independent, or even able to assist. Also, the client may require help getting to appointments on time. Consider those environmental cues and shaping techniques that may be needed to assist the client.

Identify Tasks Likely to Engage the Client

It takes time to know what interests your client, but the assessment should give some initial cues. Perhaps the person indicated that she likes to travel, or to play sports, or wants to be an artist, etc. If you know what interests your clients, you can choose tasks likely to engage them. The first tasks should have well-defined goal properties and proximal goals so that the client will quickly receive feedback and, in a short time, acquire a sense of accomplishment. As a general rule, we have found that the Frippeltration task from the Thinkin' Things™ Collection 2 software program and Venn from the Math Arena™ software program engage many adults for the first one or two sessions. People are always pleased to improve their memory and reasoning, and the tasks have many levels, accommodating clients with a wide range of skill levels. It is an excellent way to assess and teach mouse and computer skills, ability to stay on task, cognitive style, processing speed, and working memory. The treatment plan should identify several tasks that will engage the client and remediate the targeted skills.

Identify Aspects of the Learning Style That Need to Be Modified

Some clients are so dependent that they do not initiate any activity without considerable guidance. If that is the case, the treatment plan should note that the client needs to become more independent. Other clients barely tolerate the presence of the examiner. They want to do everything their own way and then get angry and stop coming when they fail. These clients need to become more comfortable accepting guidance. Some will need help dealing with auditory information, whereas others need help learning to work around others. Still others need to become less dependent on praise and feedback. Identify what about the learning style is likely to cause problems in other settings and develop a plan to modify that.

Identify Appropriate Difficulty Level

The treatment plan should indicate the level of difficulty guaranteed to provide success without being too easy. It is generally better to err on the side of being too easy, because a too easy task can be identified as being used to teach the client how to do the exercise. Tasks that are too difficult can discourage or, worse, scare off a client. The treatment plan should appreciate the client's sensitivity to any task perceived as childish. Choose tasks that the person will feel proud to be working on.

Identify Ability to Stay on Task

If the client is only able to stay on task for 5 min, then the treatment goal is to slowly increase that to 60 min (the typical length of a session). In the first week the goal would be to have the person stay on task for 10 min, and then this would be progressively increased over the next 2 months. For some clients, a goal is to have them attend and arrive on time regularly. The treatment plan might note the use of attendance certificates given weekly or less frequently.

Identify Need for Computer Training

If the person needs training to use the computer and mouse, the treatment plan needs to specify how this will be done. Some people benefit from an introduction to the computer or simple exercises to improve mouse control. Many others pick up the skill as they start the various exercises.

Identify Frequency and Duration of the Sessions

Cognitive remediation must take place at least twice a week if it is going to be effective. Greater frequency seems to be associated with faster improvement. If it is impossible to schedule a client for two or more sessions per week, then it is better to wait until the person is able to do so. The only time to have once-a-week sessions is when the person is phasing out of treatment. The duration of the sessions varies according to the ability of the client to work productively. It is better to have a short session that leaves the client feeling positive and wanting to come back than to have a long frustrating session. Some people can only tolerate 15 min the first week but invariably start to stay longer in the sessions that follow. Set aside blocks of 30 min, and stop the session at a point when the person has had an experience of success and before she starts to tire. For most clients we recommend 60-min slots, with 50 min devoted to exercises and 10 min for organizing and making notes. It is best to schedule sessions so that there is a period of 1–2 days in between sessions. The question often arises, "How many sessions are required?" The answer to this question depends on the goals of treatment. If the goal is to improve cognitive skills *and* help the person become sufficiently self-confident and comfortable with learning that they can move into mainstream learning/vocational situations, then 6 months to a year of twice a week sessions is likely necessary. If the goal is simply to make improvement on tests of cognitive functions, far less time may be needed. We advocate for the more comprehensive goal and therefore the longer course of treatment.

Identify the Software to Be Used

The treatment plan should indicate which software is going to be used to target the identified areas of cognitive deficit. In the first few sessions, the emphasis should be on engaging the client, and software should be picked that will be viewed as interesting and obviously relevant to their goals. That is not the time to do tasks that will be experienced as frustrating or tedious. Chapter 4 on software analysis provides guidance on choosing software.

Identify the Appropriate Group Learning Environment

Consider factors like age, sex, and educational and vocational backgrounds of the other clients when enrolling someone in a group. For example, one woman in a group of five men might be difficult, or one 18-year-old man in a group of five middle-aged women would not be a comfortable fit that enhances group process. It is a good idea to pair reserved and outgoing people, because having a roomful of loud, irritable, and highly distractible people can be counterproductive.

Although the goal is for the client to be able to work with six other people in the same room, some clients are so easily distracted and needy that they may initially require highly individualized attention. This is most often true of behaviorally disruptive adolescents or psychiatrically unstable inpatients, but individual or two-client sessions should not be necessary more than 2–3 times. It is also possible to pair the less functional person with higher-functioning, more independent clients who can tolerate the CRS spending considerable time with someone else. When devising the treatment plan, some note should be made of whether the client can work in a group setting and, if so, the type of clients she would likely work best with.

General Tips on Treatment Planning in the Beginning Phase of Treatment

The main goals in the first 2–3 weeks of treatment are to get the client engaged, to become acquainted with the cognitive style and needs of the client, and to do some formal assessment. The best way to get a client engaged is to foster intrinsic motivation, and that is done with several techniques. One technique is to provide exercises that are engaging, contextualized, personalized, and allow the client to feel control over the learning process. Another technique is to foster a sense of belonging to The Learning Center. Intrinsic motivation and self-determination in learning are increased by a sense of belonging to a group that values learning, by a sense of perceived competence to do socially valued activities (like learning), and by the experience of autonomy or control over the learning process. Self-perceived competence will come if the right difficulty level and right tasks are chosen. Autonomy and control are gained by showing the user options in the software, by having the client fill out session ratings and logs, and by encouraging as much independence as possible in deciding which of the tasks (of the ones shown by the CRS) she will work on. Belonging is slower to come, but pairing the client with another client or a senior client mentor helps in the beginning. Later, participation in program activities like the newsletter or assignment of jobs in The Learning Center, like analyzing and rating new software or producing the weekly certificates, will foster a sense of belonging.

Using Task Approach Analysis to Guide Treatment Planning Throughout the Treatment Phases

Treatment planning relies on an ongoing assessment of the client's strengths and weaknesses. One way to understand clients' cognitive impairment is through formal assessment, but repeated formal assessment is impractical once treatment commences. Another method is to observe how they approach tasks, because this will indicate not only how they are likely to approach tasks in other environments like work or home, but it will also reveal their cognitive or neuropsychological profile. Although there is often a best or most efficient way to do something, there are an endless number of paths a person can take toward each end. Many of the individuals utilizing The Learning Center will not automatically use the more effective or efficient strategy when completing a task. A close look at what they are doing and how they are thinking about the task can yield some very useful information about the client and may guide intervention within the context of cognitive remediation as well as in the context of the individual's overall goals.

Understanding someone's cognitive profile is really another way of saying, in what way does this person navigate life, handle novel situations, and make decisions, and what are the cognitive factors/behaviors that prevent the person from performing optimally in all situations (i.e., what is the underlying neuropsychological profile)? Within the context of the activities engaged in during cognitive remediation sessions, much of this real-world information can be gathered through careful observation. The following case examples illustrate this concept.

Case Example 1

Mr. W is a 42-year-old man diagnosed with schizoaffective disorder, who would like to return to work. Mr. W is poorly related, emotionally flat, and very quiet. He last worked at a job restocking a warehouse, but he lost the job because his boss said he was too slow. A formal neuropsychological assessment revealed above average problem solving (79th percentile) and visual memory (84th percentile), average range reaction time (33rd percentile), and attention/concentration in the deficient range (2nd percentile). Based on this, the treatment plan initially focused on attention. When he worked at the task Frippletration, another problem became apparent. In Frippletration, a memory activity that entails uncovering two pictures at a time with the goal of finding all the matching pairs on the board, Mr. W was fairly successful at making matches but so slow that he had difficulty staying on task. The CRS asked if he had a strategy to finding matches, and he explained that he envisioned the board in four quadrants, with each quadrant containing four items, which he mentally numbered one through four (see Figure 6.1 for an illustration).

This technique helped Mr. W to remember where he saw clues. He approached the task by uncovering all the ones (the upper-left item of each quadrant) first. Then he would uncover all the twos (each of the upper-right items within each quadrant). By using this system, he was able to remember the location of items based on quadrant and position within that quadrant. He was actually spontaneously using a memory strategy, albeit an overly elaborate one, given the task. In fact, the

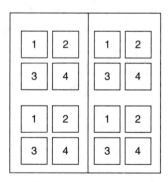

Figure 6.1
Mr. W's Quadrant Strategy

strategy was so cumbersome that it slowed him down and he lost focus. This task analysis suggested that his idiosyncratic approach to tasks, which tended toward compartmentalizing things rather than viewing the "big picture," might be contributing to his slow performance in employment settings.

The CRS used this information to adapt the treatment plan to include tasks of estimation and processing speed. She introduced Mr. W to Budget Breaker from Math Arena™. Mr. W was also encouraged to adjust the timer and challenge himself with requirements for faster response times.

Case Example 2

Mr. Y is a 53-year-old man with a diagnosis of schizophrenia, who is personable, and has the goal of independent living. Brief neuropsychological testing indicated impairment in problem solving (10th percentile), visual memory (4th percentile), and in attention/concentration (5th percentile). Based on this assessment, he was first given the previously mentioned task, Frippeltration, to improve his memory and attention. A task approach analysis revealed that this would not, however, help his memory. Mr. Y seemed to take a very long time to complete each board. His technique was to uncover the first clue on the upper left corner of the board, and then proceed to uncover all the other clues, in linear sequence, until he discovered its mate. He would then proceed to the next clue and repeat this sequential linear process until the board was cleared. His strategy was very organized, but inefficient. It also prevented any memory training, because Mr. Y was not attempting to remember any of the items he uncovered en route to finding his target. His chosen technique, although very time-consuming, was a compensatory strategy because he was reluctant to rely on his visual memory, which was poor. This strategy also reflected his linear thinking and poor working memory.

Mr. Y's strategy on this game gives many clues about how he may function if living independently. It is evident that he is not someone who can juggle many facts or tasks. He needs to complete one thing at a time. In complex situations that demand adapting strategies based on feedback, he would likely have difficulty with flexible thinking.

Based on this task approach analysis, the CRS decided that it would be best to discourage Mr. Y from doing Frippeltration, which only appeared to be reinforcing his rigid cognitive style. Instead he was given Stocktopus, which requires strategic thinking and enhances working memory. Because it progresses very slowly from easy to difficult levels, Mr. Y could ease his way into the challenging exercises that require more flexible thinking.

Case Example 3

Ms. C is a 27-year-old, socially reserved woman with schizophrenia, who would like to complete her Associate's degree at community college, but has found it difficult to manage her time and complete assignments. Brief neuropsychological testing indicated impairments in problem solving (8th percentile), verbal memory (4th percentile), and in attention/concentration (5th percentile). Given her recovery goals and the evidenced impairment on testing, the CRS gave her the task Fripplehouse, which requires one to use verbal clues to accurately place creatures ("Fripples") with assorted features (color, items of clothing, etc.) into their designated "homes." Ms. C initially could only hold on to one clue at a time, and had difficulty integrating information. Initially, this task is simple in that each home is clearly labeled with a clue as to who lives there (e.g., "A red, striped Fripple lives here."). Ms. C evidenced some difficulty on these easy levels because of her poor attention to detail when reading. For example, when asked to read aloud the clue, "The Fripple below wears a hat," Ms. C read, "The Fripple wears a hat," and proceeded to place the Fripple with the hat into the home that contained that clue, not the home below where it actually belonged. This tendency to miss words when reading became much less frequent when she was reminded periodically to reread clues and to double-check her work. However, Ms. C had difficulty of a completely different sort on more advanced levels in which she had to integrate two or more clues to figure out where Fripples lived. In these instances, Ms. C's poor working memory and cognitive rigidity hindered her performance a great deal. It was evident that she had difficulty "holding" more than one clue in mind as she searched for the applicability of additional clues. For example, Ms. C read a clue that said, "All Westside Fripples wear hats." She then proceeded to fill those houses without regard to other variables. When the CRS reminded her to check if any other rules exist that would help to determine the exact location of each hat-wearing Fripple, she nodded in recognition and searched the board. However, she was unable to mentally maintain the hat clue as she read other clues. When she stumbled upon a second clue stating that "all top floor Fripples are green," she began to place green Fripples on the top floor. She not only forgot to keep the original clue in mind, but she lost sight of the immediate goal of placing the Westside Fripples in their respective homes.

This task approach analysis confirmed the presence of multiple deficits found on neuropsychological assessment and indicated that Ms. C would benefit from tasks that exercise working memory, attention, and problem solving. The CRS decided that as a next step she would show Ms. C the task Venn from Math Arena™, because this exercise has a proximal, well-defined goal and requires that one simultaneously hold in mind three sorting principles.

Case Example 4

Ms. L is a 62-year-old female diagnosed with schizophrenia, whose goal is to find employment. A brief neuropsychological assessment revealed severely impaired reaction time (<1st percentile) and attention/concentration (2nd percentile). Ms. L was difficult to work with at first. She seemed bored with tasks, did not seem excited to learn, and did not take any initiative in selecting programs or planning her session. In fact, she did not seem to take the initiative to do very much at all. Although she was fully capable of loading a CD and starting a program, she would invariably sit, facing her computer, with the CD-ROM disk lying on the desk next to her. Without prompting she would stay in that state for an extended period of time. When asked about this she would respond with "umm," or "oh, should I start?" Similar situations would arise when she completed programs. Whereas most clients would know what to do or alert the CRS that they were finished, she would sit passively until approached.

While it was evident that Ms. L had difficulty initiating activity, it was also clear that she had difficulty recalling the sequence of steps required to accomplish a task such that repeated prompting was necessary for her to complete such routine tasks as loading a CD-ROM and starting a program. Initially, asking her guiding questions like "What do you think is the first thing you have to do to get started working on this program?" or "Now that the CD-ROM is in, what is your next step?" was not helpful. It was evident that she was struggling to recall the proper sequence of steps toward achieving her desired goal. To help her, the CRS wrote on an index card three brief instructions with accompanying pictures, for starting activities. This card was placed in Ms. L's folder, and she was taught to place it by the computer at the start of the session. Through much repetition and practice (i.e., overlearning) she was able to accomplish these tasks on her own, albeit rather slowly.

Ms. L's case is also a good example of the importance of finding the right fit between task and client. For many sessions it seemed that Ms. L was only moderately interested in tasks. This persisted despite attempts to engage her in a variety of software. She tried Frippletration, Fripplehouse, Where in the U.S.A. is Carmen Sandiego?®, Math for the Real Word™, Grammar for the Real World™, Outnumbered, and Frogger. The CRS kept attempting to give her highly engaging programs that were colorful and full of action, thinking that the highly stimulating programs would hold her attention and excite her to participate. Just when nothing seemed to be working, the CRS happened to introduce Grammar Games. This is one of the least stimulating games, with no audio-visual effects, and offers no positive reinforcers until tasks are completed. One task involved reading a lengthy, singe-spaced story and correcting certain highlighted grammatically incorrect words. This was an untimed task in which there was no penalty for slow performance. Ms. L took to this task immediately and commented excitedly how much she was enjoying herself. At the end of the session she remarked that she felt she had learned a great deal this session, and was looking forward to using this program again next session. For Ms. L., this program was straightforward, easy to understand, and did not contain distracting elements. She found comfort in the simplicity of the task as well as the well-defined goals. The CRS used this information to find more tasks for her, like Puzzle Tanks™, another low stimulation, untimed task that promotes problem solving and flexible thinking.

Ms. L's task approach and task preferences helped inform her treatment team as to what type of employment to guide her towards. Specifically, her approach to tasks in The Learning Center makes it clear that she needs a job in which the objectives and the steps toward achieving them are well-defined. Her work environment should be low stimulation, and her job should not depend on speed. She also would succeed in a job with repetitive tasks requiring little mental flexibility. These recommendations were presented to Ms. L's team.

Sample Treatment Plans

Figures 6.2 and 6.3 show two different types of treatment plans. Feel free to use them as models when creating your own.

GOALS	STRATEGIES	PROGRAMS	PROGRESS
Improve fine motor skills	Begin with keyboard only Select programs requiring simple mouse skills Work with strengths—good vocabulary	Word Attack Spell It Deluxe Fripplehouse Frippletration	No longer sticky with keyboard Good mouse control Considerable improvement Some difficulty with "finer" motor tasks (e.g., Factory)
Increase self-esteem	Provide opportunity to use intact skills (e.g., good vocabulary, general knowledge, arithmetic) Teach other programs	Word Attack Mathblaster Math for the Real World	Teaching others has helped increase confidence and to be task focused Enjoys the opportunity to be cognitively challenged within a structured environment

Figure 6.2

Sample treatment plan #1 (Provided by Joe Gorrell, Northern Sydney Health)

GOALS	STRATEGIES	PROGRAMS	PROGRESS
Improve ability to sustain attention	Tasks requiring sustained attention—gradually increasing duration Encourage verbal regulation of behavior when losing set	Speedyracer Orangabanga Stocktopus	Some verbalization of difficult tasks Able to maintain attention to simple engaging tasks, but gets easily distracted on more complex tasks
Increase motor and processing speed	Practice on timed tasks Practice with mouse and keyboard	Leap to Complete Orangabanga	Significant improvement
Improve capacity to hold and manipulate information, working memory/ sequential thinking	Discourage trial and error approach Encourage practicing planned approach Practice dealing with complex verbal statements and problem solving tasks	Stocktopus Mathblaster (e.g., barrels, pool table) Math for the Real World Factory	Mentally planning 4–5 step trades using top down and bottom-up planning—occasional loss of set/helps to verbalize Good arithmetic skills, but needs to be reminded to stick to the task and keep it simple Gets distracted with complex math formulas Helps to ask her to rephrase the question and repeat a few times
Improve time management, initiation, finishing things, and self-monitoring	Encourage getting in and out of programs independently Encourage session planning, use of personal log, self-monitoring of time, use of clock, moving		Able to use icons and CD-ROM Some difficulty using start menu—insufficient fine motor coordination/ gets distracted by something interesting and ends up in another program

Figure 6.2 *continued*

Problem	Long Range Goal	Objective	Intervention
1. Poor attention and concentration	Client will maintain goal-directed behavior in vocational settings	Client will increase time on cognitive exercise from 10 to 30 min	Use of engaging software programs to promote goal-directed behavior and concentration (e.g., twice weekly sessions using Math Arena, Frippeltration, Orangabanga, Grammar for the Real World)
2. Disorganization	Client will approach tasks in an orderly sequence and demonstrate flexibility in problem solving in order to enhance vocational functioning	Client will demonstrate independent use of activities that rely on information processing, planning, organization	Use of software programs to maximize problem solving (e.g., twice weekly sessions using The Factory, Puzzle Tanks, Stocktopus, and Carmen World).

Figure 6.3

Sample treatment plan #2.

Remediation of Attention and Working Memory Deficits

There are a few programs available that were designed to improve attention in individuals with head injury. For example, the Captain's Log software from Brain Train® is a highly structured program that provides good feedback and tracking of progress, and includes tasks that focus exclusively on attention. Instructional features to enhance intrinsic motivation and engagement are not featured, but clients who are committed to improving attention may choose to work on these tasks. For most clients, we have found that there are other highly engaging educational programs that were not designed to improve attention but nevertheless have a beneficial impact. For example, Leap to Complete is an exercise from the Spell It® Deluxe software program that is excellent at fostering visual scanning, vigilance, working memory, processing speed, and reaction time, all within the context of an exercise that improves spelling. A number of exercises in Math Arena™ (e.g. Mistake Catcher, Quick Change) are also excellent at remediating attention. Positscience (www.Positscience.com) is a company that is developing software to remediate attention in schizophrenia and dementia, and some of their activities include motivationally enhancing components.

Neuropsychological and Educational Approach to Cognitive Remediation (NEAR) uses a variety of drill and practice attention exercises within multiple learning contexts. NEAR also promotes metacognitive awareness and self-monitoring of attention and vigilance through feedback and discussion of specific examples of a client's cognitive performance. This discussion is casual so that the client does not feel attacked, and may consist of a sentence or two commenting about the client's cognitive style. The cognitive rehabilitation specialist could, for example, say, *"Everyone has a cognitive style. I notice that you focus on many things at once."* Gently encourage the client to become aware of his own style, and to consider examples of attention functioning from situations outside The Learning Center. It is often wise to first discuss how a cognitive style is adaptive before remarking on the maladaptive features. Thus, if the CRS asks, *"How does it work for you when you focus on many things at once?"* the client may spontaneously remark, *"I guess I don't get bored that way, but my supervisor says that I should slow down and focus on one thing at a time."*

Attention remediation typically begins with structured visual scanning and basic selective attention exercises, and then progressively increases in difficulty as exercises are added that challenge divided attention, working memory, and sustained attention. Attention exercises are presented using a variety of learning contexts, knowledge domains, and stimulus modalities (i.e., visual, auditory, verbal, and nonverbal). Even when the focus of the remediation sessions has shifted to problem solving, attention is still periodically targeted for intervention. Sometimes, when clients experience psychiatric setbacks, they find it helpful to return to the basic attention exercises.

Remediation of Memory Deficits

The ability to remember the time of an appointment requires that information has been attended to, encoded, stored, and then retrieved. Problems can occur at any juncture in this series of steps, with resultant poor memory. Perhaps because memory is a complex skill, it is best helped by a comprehensive treatment strategy that targets multiple cognitive skills and does not just drill and practice mnemonic techniques. Because memory deficits can sometimes be partly caused by reduced attention, the CRS should discuss with clients the importance of attention and intent to remember during situations when later recall of information will be important. Increased attention, verbal repetition, and note taking are techniques that make intuitive sense to clients. Other compensatory strategies to teach are time-spaced repetitive rehearsal of new material, making explicit connections to prior knowledge or experience, and "chunking" new material into obvious categories. Teaching these simple encoding and compensatory techniques can improve memory and cognitive organization.

There are environmental aids that can also be presented to clients who report difficulty remembering their keys, or scheduling or returning phone calls. Encourage the use of alarm clocks, organizers, key hooks, Post-it® notes, and checklists. These are all good memory aids that many clients have never learned to use. Promote intrinsic motivation and independent use of external aids by engaging the client in the personalized selection of a calendar or agenda that is appropriate for his current activities. By assisting the client in the initial use of the agenda, and by spending several minutes in each session reviewing recent agenda entries, independent use is further promoted. Also, if an agenda is used, it is important to identify a cue that will remind the person to look at the agenda. For example, the client can put his daily schedule in a pants pocket. This way, every time the client puts a hand in the pocket, he will be reminded to check the schedule.

Software programs that were designed to help memory are available, both through educational software companies and companies that design software for people with dementia. Web-based memory exercises are also available on sites developed for people who struggle with age related memory decline (e.g., www.happy-neuron.com). There are also many programs that were not designed to improve memory, but careful task analysis will indicate that they in fact tone skills needed for remembering. It is also important to ask questions that check memory. For example, the CRS can ask the client who is working on a problem solving exercise, *"What is the goal you are trying to work toward now?"* or *"What did you work on last time?"* or *"Would you mind explaining to* [another client] *how to start this program?"* These memory checks also promote self-monitoring and self-awareness, ingredients for improving insight.

Remediation of Problem Solving Deficits

Critical thinking skills, which are required to solve problems, are recognized as the most essential skills for vocational success in the twenty-first century. These skills are so essential that mainstream education now emphasizes the importance of teaching critical thinking in a way that was previously unheard of. Educational psychology has made significant contributions to the teaching of critical thinking skills, and NEAR has incorporated much of this into the treatment process. There are many critical thinking skills curriculums and educational activities that can be adapted for use in cognitive remediation programs for psychiatric patients. Furthermore, because critical thinking requires attention and working memory, in addition to the subskills that allow problem solving, we have found that many of the cognitive skills that require remediation get addressed when the focus is on problem solving. In essence, it is difficult not to be training attention, working memory, and processing speed when doing critical thinking exercises.

Effective problem solving involves a number of cognitive skills: attention; the ability to hold information in mind while considering it (working memory); the ability to identify essential problem characteristics; mental flexibility; concept formation; analogic, inductive, and deductive reasoning; decision making; initiation; planning; organization; sequencing; self-monitoring; and follow-through. NEAR explicitly teaches strategies for effective problem solving by providing individual computer-based as well as group exercises that drill and practice these various skills. Metacognitive awareness of problem solving strategies is encouraged by having the client talk about ways that he can use the skills taught in The Learning Center in everyday life.

Problem solving remediation typically begins with structured tasks that focus on basic sequencing, concept formation, identifying similarities and differences, and simple reasoning. Examples of software that provide basic problem solving exercises can be found in the Thinkin' Things™ Collection by Edmark. Introductory didactic coaching and prompting are required when clients first begin to use these (or any) programs, but once the procedures to do the exercises have been provided, clients are encouraged to practice the tasks independently. Some clients need more modeling and shaping than others in order to successfully engage in the tasks. Once the client has mastered the basic procedures and rules, continue to assist him as needed to focus on relevant problem details and organize the decision-making process.

Effective problem solving techniques are introduced incrementally in exercises that provide a variety of simulated and real contexts, and increasingly distal and complex goals. Clients are encouraged to summarize problem solving strategies in their own words and to find examples from other areas of everyday life. Be sure to continue orienting the clients to the goal, the nature of the problem, and the steps needed to reach the goal. It is also important to encourage clients to look at their results and modify their approaches if necessary. They can learn by evaluating the problem solving process.

The CRS needs to be able to choose the appropriate difficulty level for the client. In general, the difficulty levels in problem solving are determined by the following criteria:

The Degree of Temporary Memory Required to Grasp the Problem

If the client has poor working memory, he will not be able to hold information in mind long enough to understand the goal and nature of the problem. For example, Where in the World is Carmen Sandiego?® is a much more complex problem solving task than the easy levels of Fripple House, because more steps and information must be held in mind to solve the problem.

The Degree of Procedural Versus Declarative Knowledge Required

Procedural knowledge is knowledge of the steps necessary to obtain the goal. For example, in the Carmen Sandiego software, the procedures for capturing a thief are to ask witnesses for information, collect clues, fill out a warrant, and travel to the place where the thief can be arrested. For some clients, this set of procedures is too complicated and other single-step tasks are preferable. Declarative knowledge is the knowledge necessary to solve the problem. To build an airplane, one needs knowledge of aerodynamics. In the Carmen Sandiego software, knowledge of geography helps but is not necessary because the program teaches the geography. In general, NEAR tries to find programs that do not require much domain-specific knowledge, as many clients may not have it.

The Degree to Which the Goal Is Well-Defined

Most clients like structure because there is a clear-cut goal. Writing an essay about favorite foods is harder than playing Carmen Sandiego because it is never completely clear when the essay is finished. The essay could continually be edited, amended, and made better, whereas in Carmen Sandiego, you either catch the thief or you do not. For the more advanced clients, it is important to help them deal with less clear-cut goals.

Once clients have mastered several structured exercises, and have successfully implemented basic problem solving strategies, less structured, more difficult programs can be introduced. The harder programs require more initiative, information integration, organization, self-monitoring, and higher-order reasoning. Several educational software programs exist that challenge these abilities within simulated real-world or fantasy contexts, such as historical journeys, animated movie making, or small business operations.

For clients who are working to remediate higher-order problem solving and executive functioning, creating a PowerPoint presentation on a topic of interest provides an effective and challenging exercise that promotes independence, initiative, decision making, and follow-through. There are preset presentation formats on PowerPoint, available by going to "File," then "New," and then the "Autocontent Wizard," and these presentation formats provide structure to the client and teach effective communication skills. Another exercise is to work on a newsletter. Clients can engage in editing, layout, and design. A third exercise for higher-order executive functioning is to have a client critically evaluate software. Clients are always excited and pleased to be asked to look through an educational software catalog and pick the programs that look interesting. This task requires them to critically evaluate the descriptions and think about which programs are most likely to be helpful. To successfully do this exercise, the client must understand the purpose of The Learning Center, and must demonstrate sufficient critical thinking skills to evaluate the software. Once they pick the software, they can order it—most companies have a free trial period—and when it arrives they can test it. This type of activity not only improves critical thinking, it gives the client an important role in The Learning Center. Additionally, they see that their skills are valued, and are pleased to be recognized as a contributor to a valued group activity. Refer back to Chapter 4 for more information on choosing and analyzing software.

Facilitating Learning: How Involved Should the Clinician Be?

The CRS always introduces the new software he wants the client to work on, and provides instruction on the procedures to complete the task. A brief explanation of what the task helps with is also given, and then the client is left alone to explore and practice the activity. Coaching is gradually reduced as the client becomes more capable of independent task performance. One of the challenges for the CRS is to learn how to judge frustration tolerance in his clients. You do not want to step in if unnecessary because that reinforces a perception that the client is incompetent, and you don't want to allow the client to get so frustrated that he gives up. Some clients will show visible signs of frustration, leading you to think they will lose self-control, but become quite indignant if you step in, and feel that you have deprived them of a chance at success. The CRS must learn that that is the style of the client; being vocal and dramatic about frustration is just how they do things. It is best then to make a comment like, *"When you banged your hand on the table I thought you had about had it, but maybe that was just your way of really getting down to work."* The fact is that banging, cursing, and other dramatic behaviors are not socially acceptable ways to solve problems, and eventually the person will have to see that when he does that, others will either get worried and step in, depriving him of a chance to meet the goal, or will walk away and then not be around to help or appreciate the success. Other clients will quietly stare at the task, and minutes will go by without any sign of activity. Deal with this by saying something like, *"How are you doing over here? What is the goal you are working toward? What is the next step you need to do? I notice that you get really quiet sometimes. Is that your way of taking a rest when the going gets rough? You can also call me over because I am always happy to come and work on this with you."* The first step in changing that behavior is to bring awareness, and that happens when the CRS understands the situation and makes nonjudgmental observations of the behavior.

It is also important for the CRS to make statements and ask questions that help the client relate his activities in The Learning Center to real-world situations (this concept is called *generalization* and is discussed on page 13 and in Chapter 9). These kinds of comments should be given sparingly, starting around Session 4. There is no point in offering bridging comments before the client is settled into a routine and has sufficient mastery of the task to develop some perspective on the overall goal. When someone is first learning a task, he is usually so focused on acquiring the procedures or mastering the task that he may not be able to appreciate the links between the task activity and real-life activities. Furthermore, clients vary in their ability to think in the abstract, which might make the task of bridging more challenging for the CRS and the client.

Guided Questions Strategy

Following are examples of questions you can ask clients in order to facilitate optimal performance when they are working on tasks in The Learning Center.

Broad Questions

These are the types of guiding questions to start with if a client appears to be struggling with a task:

1. What is your goal in this activity?

2. What do you think is the next step?

3. What are the different ways you can meet your goal?

4. I noticed you did X, do you think it worked well? If not, say, "Let's go back and try something else."

Specific Questions

If broad questions fail to guide the client, ask more specific questions, such as (example questions 1–4 are for Carmen Sandiego games):

1. Where do you have to travel?

2. Where did you come from? Where are you going next?

3. What are your choices and options when you arrive at a new city?

4. Do you need to get more information about where the thief went or about what they look like?

5. What do you know about all the purple fripples? (for the Fripple House software)

Figure 7.1 shows the steps of the guided questions strategy.

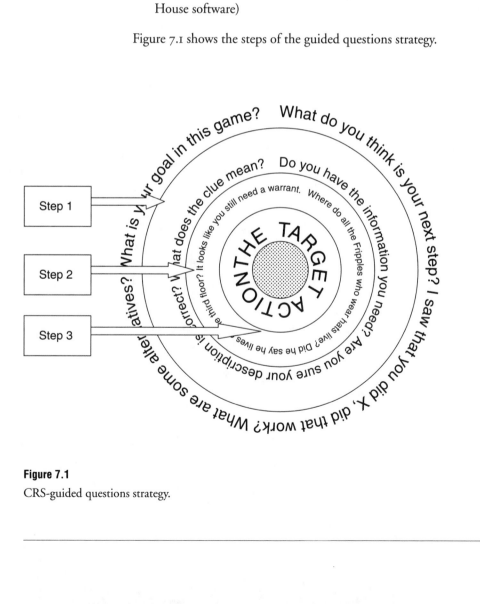

Figure 7.1
CRS-guided questions strategy.

In addition to asking questions to facilitate optimal performance of tasks, you also may wish to ask clients how the activities they are working on translate into real life:

1. How do you think doing this activity will help you outside The Learning Center?

2. Are the things you are doing in this activity similar to things you do in real life?

3. You told me you had problems with your memory; do you think this activity might help you? How so?

Chapter 8 *Phases of Treatment*

The Beginning Phase of Treatment

Session 1

Before the session begins, make a folder for each client by stapling the Software I Have Learned To Use at The Learning Center form to the left inside page of a file folder and the Individual Session Log to the right inside page of the folder (copies of these forms for your use are provided in the appendix). Bring this folder to the session, and after greeting the client provide some orienting comments that include some reference to the intake appointment and the goals discussed there, and recollection of the software tried at that meeting. Encourage clients to be collaborators in the learning process by offering them the chance to ask questions, give suggestions, and provide feedback. Show them the folders you have made up for them, and explain that in the beginning of every session each client gets her folder and chooses an activity from the list of activities on the Software I Have learned to Use at The Learning Center form. Show clients where the activities/software are kept. Explain that after every session they will complete the Individual Session Log in their folders and that the folders thus serve as a document of what they have done at The Learning Center. Ask them to write their names on their folders and to enter the name of the first activity you have shown/will show them. Then help them get to work on the task, and once they are settled in, leave them to work independently.

If a client has little experience with a computer, provide her with an initial introduction to hardware and software. Keep the introduction brief, because most people learn best by actually using the computer. An introduction could go as follows:

> *The computer is made up of several parts. The box here that looks like a TV screen is called a monitor. It is here that pictures and information are displayed. The box here is called the systems unit and that is where the main electronic circuits can be found, and is the "brain" of the computer. This is the power button, which is used to turn the computer on. If the light is on, that means the computer is already turned on and there is no need to press it. If the light is off, you can press that button to turn on the computer. In front, here, there is a rectangular button. Push it. See, a drawer opens up, and that is where the CD-ROM goes. The CD-ROMs we use here look just like the ones you might use to listen to music. Although these look the same, these contain information that the computer uses, which could be music, pictures, or even movies. Many of the exercises you will be doing are on CD-ROM disks. Last week you worked on this one. Let's put it in. Remember, whenever you put in a disk, it is important to make sure that the writing is always facing up and that the disk is resting correctly in the tray (give them the disk to put in). Push this button here to close the drawer. See how the program starts automatically? Not all programs start automatically; when you get one that has to be started, I will show you how to do that. Before we get started on this program, let me show you how the keyboard and mouse work.*

Spend several minutes demonstrating the mouse and keyboard. The Windows Notepad or Control Panel mouse settings can be used to allow temporary practice of keyboard input and mouse drag and click technique. The concept of moving the mouse and using single and double clicks should be understood. It can also be helpful to review the screen display and show how to scan the screen with the windshield wiper technique, that is, moving the eyes back and forth across the screen.

At that point, start the client on a program, something like Frippletration, a highly structured task with a clear goal that can be completed in a brief time. Introduce the task by saying something like this: *"We will be using several software programs to improve your concentration, attention, memory, and thinking skills."* Then proceed to describe and explain the specific task chosen. For example, if the chosen starting task is

Frippletration, describe the task as a matching activity that improves memory. You may wish to say something like the following:

In this activity you have to use your memory to make matches. Do you see these boxes? Well, they are hiding things. You can reveal what is behind each box by clicking on it with the mouse. Why don't you try that? OK, now you have to click on a second box. If the item behind that box matches the other one you opened, you will have your first match. If not, both boxes will cover themselves up again. Part of your job is to remember what is behind the boxes you open. Let's keep going and see if we can make a match.

Sit slightly behind the client so that you can assist as needed but not intrude. Make remarks that guide without telling the person what to do. Provide periodic positive feedback that is specific. Thus, instead of saying something vague like *"Great!"* tell them what was great: *"I like the way you stick with the task even when it is hard,"* or *"You seem to have really got the hang of using a mouse,"* or *"It looked like you were working hard to remember, and when you did that you were successful."* Some clients will look constantly to you for feedback, and you should gratify that need for validation, at least in the beginning. However, you can train them to recognize a simple nonverbal gesture, like a thumbs-up, as a sign that you appreciate their work. Of course, the eventual goal is for them to be self-confident enough not to need constant validation.

For most clients, working on two tasks is enough for the first session. When you notice that the client is less attentive or frustrated with the first activity, suggest that it is time to stop. Ask how she found the task and if she would like to continue working on it another day. Offer to show the client the second task, another one with proximal goals that can be finished quickly. If the client seems ready to leave for the day, have her fill out the activity sheet. Review the schedule and time for the next session. Some clients, especially those with poor attention and frustration tolerance, will want to essentially flip through every software program they can find, taking it off the screen as soon as it comes up. Hopefully, your initial assessment will have alerted you to this potential and you will only have two programs available for them to try the first session. With these clients it is important to start with a program that is easy to use and will give constant and immediate feedback. These are the clients who do better with brief sessions in the beginning.

You will find the following guidelines helpful when presenting didactic instruction to clients in the first session:

- Explanations of new material or procedures should be succinct, presented in an organized sequence and with a level of detail and vocabulary appropriate to the client's cognitive ability.

- Presentations of new information should be combined with repeated demonstrations and opportunities for practice.

- Some clients find it helpful to take notes. For example, they might write on an index card the procedures for starting a computer and opening a program. They can then pull this card from their file at the start of every session.

- Move at a pace that is comfortable for the client. Watch the nonverbal cues, and make sure more time is spent having the client learn actively rather than passively.

- Explain to clients using the more elementary activities with proximal goals that they should do at least two different tasks like that in any session so as to practice their skills in different contexts. For example, do not let someone work on any one Math Arena activity for the whole session. If the client is working on a more complex activity like Carmen Sandiego or Hot Dog Stand, they may use the whole session.

Over the course of the first six remediation sessions, three or four different software exercises should be introduced that will target the identified cognitive deficits. Start with the more structured tasks, and slowly add those with more complexity. In any given session, the client chooses which of the activities on the list in her folder she wants to work on—provided she works on enough activities. Sometimes a session can end by asking the client what she would like to work on first the next time. The client can write down the activity in her folder to remind herself at the next session. It is okay if a client decides to change her mind and start with something different than she had originally planned; the point is that the client is starting to take initiative. Try to encourage the client to verbalize her reasons for wanting to start with a given program as this promotes self-awareness of learning style. By allowing the client control over nonessential aspects of the remediation process, as in choosing which program to work on next, intrinsic motivation and autonomy are promoted. Although every client requires her own treatment plan that guides the selection of software, it is useful for the beginning cognitive rehabilitation specialist (CRS) to have some sense of what order to introduce software and generally how to structure the first few sessions. The basic template shown in Table 8.1 can serve as a guide until you feel more comfortable structuring sessions on your own. You may also find it helpful to use Table 8.2 which provides a list of appropriate software for specific cognitive skills.

Table 8.1 Basic Template for the First Few Sessions of Treatment

Session 1	Introduce the client to The Learning Center. Explain the mission of the program (i.e., to improve thinking skills/work toward goals) and what is expected of the client (i.e., to keep appointments, to respect the equipment and peers).
	Show the client where her folder will be stored. Explain the sign-in/activity log sheet.
	Introduce client to computer and practice with mouse and keyboard.
	Introduce client to one or two software titles. Frippletration from Thinkin' Things™ Collection 2 and Venn from Math Arena™ are good titles to start with.
	Always start at the *easiest* level. You can always adjust the level to suit the client if the initial level proves to be too easy. It is better that the client has an easy success than a quick failure, which could cause her to be reluctant to continue.
Session 2	Depending on the client, it may be necessary to reiterate some basic computer instruction, and some continued practice with the mouse and computer navigation may be necessary. It may also be necessary to remind the client to get her folder and sign the activity sheet.
	Return to software introduced in Session 1. Resume at the level achieved at the end of the first session.
	For many clients, this session is spent working on the same programs as in Session 1. However, for others (e.g., those who dislike the first program/found the first program too difficult/are easily bored) it may be prudent to introduce another task, for example, Combo Cubes from Math Arena™.

continued

Table 8.1 Basic Template for the First Few Sessions of Treatment *continued*

Session 3   If the previous two sessions were spent working on two activities, you can now offer the client an opportunity to work on a third program. If the client wishes to continue with the first two programs, allow her to continue.

Use observation and task approach analysis from the first two sessions to choose cognitive skills to target with another software exercise. Table 8.2 lists software titles categorized by the basic cognitive skills they teach.

Session 4   By the end of this session, the client should have been exposed to at least three software titles.

In this, and the sessions to follow, you must continually evaluate the client's performance, task approach, frustration tolerance, and ability to learn, and monitor the difficulty levels of the software the client is using as well as the appropriateness of new titles.

Table 8.2 Software for Specific Cognitive Skills

Skills	Software	Level of difficulty
Problem solving, deductive reasoning, inductive reasoning, attention to detail	Frippleshop	Easy
	Puzzle Tanks™	Moderate
	Fripple House	Easy to difficult
	Stocktopus	Easy to difficult
	Outnumbered	Moderate (requires motor skills)
	Carmen Sandiego USA/World	USA is easier than World; Both range in levels of difficulty from moderate to difficult
	Venn from Math Arena™	Easy to difficult
	Cross Country USA	Moderate to difficult
	The Factory	Easy to difficult
	Hot Dog Stand	Difficult
	Math for the Real World™	Moderate
	Grammar for the Real World™	Moderate
Visual/auditory memory	Frippletration	Easy to difficult
	Carmen USA/Carmen World	USA is easier than World; Both range in levels of difficulty from moderate to difficult
	Cross Country USA	Moderate to difficult

continued

Skills	Software	Level of difficulty
Working memory/sequencing	Carmen USA/Carmen World	USA is easier than World; Both range in levels of difficulty from moderate to difficult
	Outnumbered	Moderate
	Stocktopus	Easy to difficult
	Math Arena™	Easy to difficult
	The Factory	Easy to difficult
	Fripple House	Easy to difficult
	Grammar for the Real World™ (selected exercises)	Moderate
	Math for the Real World™ (selected exercises)	Moderate
Attention/concentration	Word Attack	Easy to difficult
	Maze Game	Easy to difficult
	Frippletration	Easy to difficult
	Math for the Real World™	Moderate
	Math Arena™	Easy to difficult
Processing speed/response time/hand–eye coordination	Leap to Complete	Easy to difficult
	Frogger	Moderate to difficult
	Outnumbered	Use timer to adjust processing speed and the easy-to-difficult bar to adjust problem solving level
	Math Arena™	Use timer to adjust processing speed and the easy-to-difficult bar to adjust problem solving level

Table 8.3 is a sample session schedule showing how to introduce eight software activities that address the following four basic skill areas:

■ Memory

■ Attention

■ Problem solving

■ Processing speed

This schedule may not be ideal for every client but will work well for the client who adjusts readily to the cognitive remediation program.

Table 8.3 Sample Cognitive Remediation Session Schedule (18 Sessions)

Session number	Software programs to introduce
1	Venn (Math Arena™), Frippeltration (Thinkin' Things™ Collection 2)
2	
3	Stocktopus (Thinkin' Things™ Collection 3)
4	
5	Frippleshop or Fripple House* (Thinkin' Things™ Collection 2)
6	
7	Combo Cubes (Math Arena™)
8	
9	
10	The Factory
11	
12	
13	Grammar or Math for the Real World™ or Zoombinis™*
14	
15	
16	Where in the USA is Carmen Sandiego?®
17	
18	
19	

* Choose one depending on client's skill level.

The Middle Phase of Treatment

Once the client is engaged in the learning process, she has entered the middle phase of treatment. This is the phase when the most cognitive growth occurs. The client has settled in, is familiar with the routines and procedures, and is, so to speak, ready to get to work. Emotional and learning style issues still interfere with productivity and learning, but clients are motivated and more receptive to feedback; they are excited about learning and more purposeful in their quest for knowledge.

What are the signs that the clients are engaged? They come regularly to sessions, and if they cannot attend, they notify the CRS ahead of time. They arrive punctually and look irritated or crestfallen if all the seats are full. For those clients with persistent memory or organizational problems who have trouble remembering sessions, they are actively working on developing/using techniques to assist attendance. Some clients stop by at unscheduled times to see if they can come in and work (which is acceptable if a computer is free, the CRS is available, and the client is on time for her appointment.) When the clients come in, they seem eager to get to work. They are starting to show signs of independence—they spontaneously get their folders and look over the programs they want to use. When they are at work they show a positive attitude about learning, are focused and serious, and show more awareness of cognitive style and learning process. Clients who were rigid and tense in the beginning become more willing to explore and try new activities; clients who were unable to stay on task now focus for longer periods of time.

The CRS should by this point have a good sense of the cognitive and learning style issues that compromise adaptive functioning. In the middle phase of treatment, clients are more settled, so it is possible to see the stylistic and emotional factors that disrupt cognitive functioning. Also, the CRS should have a better sense of what interests each client and her talents and strengths. Armed with this knowledge, the CRS can better guide the learning process and make sure it is a positive, productive experience. Clients should be shown exercises that will help them, and continue to excite and interest them. As in the beginning phase, ongoing monitoring of competency level and encouragement of independence continue to be essential.

Case Example

Maria is a 42-year-old with major depression who was referred to The Learning Center because of memory difficulties. She had trouble remembering appointments, remembering where she put her agenda, or notes she had written to remind her of things. She has a high school diploma and worked in clerical jobs until depression and homelessness dominated her life. Maria likes to read popular novels, and is a very quiet person who avoids eye contact and conversation. She wants to work but has been fired from jobs because she cannot remember information told to her. Maria's assessment indicated average intellectual ability, with impairments in processing speed, attention, reaction time, working memory, and especially in memory.

Maria rapidly settled into the routines and liked working on programs with clear-cut goals. She showed patience and a good ability to stay on task. She asked for extra sessions and arrived punctually. Maria was given exercises to improve her attention, processing speed, organizational ability, and working memory. She demonstrated ever-improving problem solving strategies but persistent poor memory. For example, the CRS noticed that although she knew she had to capture the thief in the game Carmen, and knew the procedures for doing this, she never remembered what the thief had stolen. The CRS started to make a point of saying, "I will ask you later about this," in order to prime her to remember. Throughout the sessions, the CRS would ask questions to prime Maria's memory. They talked about strategies for remembering. Some specific computer-based memory exercises were also done.

Although Maria worked independently, the CRS noticed that she constantly looked for feedback. Her approach to the tasks seemed insecure and anxious. She would do something and then look for approval. It was felt that this anxious style was also interfering with remembering. In order to help increase Maria's self-confidence, the following plan was developed.

1. When the CRS gave verbal feedback, it was specific positive feedback, for example, "When you scanned the entire page for clues, you were able to find the answer," as opposed to general feedback like "Great."

2. The CRS made a nonverbal sign of recognition when she was busy with another client and Maria looked up for feedback.

3. At the end of the week, the CRS gave Maria a certificate listing her accomplishments.

4. After 2 weeks of receiving certificates, Maria was asked to be the person who helped create the certificates for other clients. The CRS would give her the information, and she would type up the certificates and print them. Maria enjoyed this. She liked learning to use the computer and made some good suggestions about certificate formats. She was given a role that gave her some control

over feedback, and she was making an important contribution to The Learning Center.

After 5 weeks, Maria stopped looking to the CRS for feedback. She became more secure and sure of herself. She practiced multiple tasks that require retention of verbal information as well as organization of information. Her memory improved to the point that she was able to travel independently, and she did not need people to call and remind her about appointments. Scores on memory tests improved to the average range.

The End Phase of Treatment

There comes a point in treatment when the client seems to have made gains in her cognitive functioning, is more independent, and seems ready to move on. This is the time when retesting on the baseline cognitive measures seems in order. The client is often eager to be retested, senses that she has made gains, and looks forward to see if the test results confirm her impression. The test results can guide decisions. Perhaps there is more work to be done. Alternatively, it may be time to move on.

For many people, The Learning Center is not a place they want to leave. It is therefore helpful to transition clients into the next phase of their life. For some, this transition can take months; for others, they start to engage in new activities, and somehow, despite plans to come back and have sessions, they do not have time. The end phase of treatment is also the time to deal with lingering emotional-social issues that interfere with optimal cognitive success.

One way to facilitate the transition to new programs is to have a tiered system in The Learning Center where clients can move from full-time client to assistant. There are many jobs in The Learning Center that can be done by clients, and clients benefit from participating in valued roles. One job might be to explain tasks to new clients, another job might be to edit the newsletter, and another might be to assist with clerical tasks. Jobs should be carefully chosen to fit the skills of the particular client.

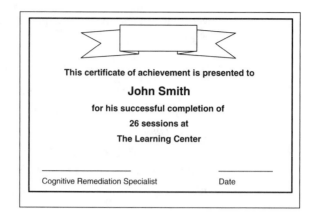

This certificate of achievement is presented to

John Smith

for his successful completion of

26 sessions at

The Learning Center

_____   _____

Cognitive Remediation Specialist   Date

Figure 8.1
Certificate of completion.

Other clients will start job training and may only have time for one session a week. It is important for clients to know that they are always welcome to come back for "booster" sessions, even if they graduate. They should also know that the CRS is interested to hear how they are doing. Perhaps they want to submit a note to the newsletter; perhaps they would like to come back and talk to the group about their experiences.

A graduation ceremony can be a good closure experience, and clients attach great meaning to gaining a certificate of completion (see Figure 8.1 for an example). Other staff, clients, and the graduating client's guests should be invited. Let the clients help with the ceremony. Perhaps they would like to choose the cake and drinks. Give time for people to make toasts and take pictures. Be sure to post the event on the bulletin board.

Case Example (Maria continued)

Maria showed improvement in all her test scores, and most importantly, she felt better able to cope with everyday tasks. She was proud of her accomplishment and was receiving positive feedback from her caseworker, who also noticed the improvement. At The Learning

Center, she was working quite independently. She had tried all the programs and gotten to the top level on some of them. She was asking about what else she could do, hoping that there was more to be accomplished there. She was starting to look at jobs and had put in an application. Nevertheless, she did not seem quite ready for that transition.

The CRS noticed that Maria had very poor people skills. She did not like to talk to other clients, would barely answer if asked questions, and seemed uncomfortable in the group. Her preference was to sit uninterrupted at the computer. During the bridging group, she would often turn to the computer, as if to start working on it. She also seemed quite uncomfortable with tasks that did not have a clear-cut goal. Maria's cognitive skills had improved greatly, but her social skills were interfering with adaptive functioning. To deal with these problems, the following plan was developed:

1. The CRS started to make nonjudgmental comments to Maria about her clear preference to work quietly. They talked about how she handles work environments where colleagues are talkative.

2. Maria was given Grammar for The Real World™ to work on because it has simulations of different bosses and Maria could see how she responded to their styles. She was also given exercises that were less directed, like writing an essay or doing a web search.

3. Maria was given the role of secretary in the group. Although there was concern that the role of secretary would shield her from confronting her social anxiety, it was felt that the comfort she would derive from having a purpose, and having a pad of paper to look at, might enable her to feel comfortable enough to participate. She was given a socially appropriate and productive way to deal with her anxiety.

4. Given her good organizational and clerical skills, and the initiative she had shown in trying out new software, Maria was asked if she would like to work a couple of hours a week as a paid assistant in the program. She was given jobs where she had to interact with people around clerical issues.

5.   The CRS spoke in team meeting about the need for Maria to get more social skills training.

Maria worked as an assistant for several months, continued sessions twice a week, and during that time also started to look for jobs. The whole team worked with her to help find an appropriate placement. She was accepted into a job-training program to work on data entry, a job that suited her disposition. Maria graduated, less anxious, more confident, better able to remember, still isolative, but more aware of the ways she could contribute to social interactions.

Chapter 9　　*Bridging Groups*

One of the greatest challenges to any skills-acquisition training program is the transfer of skills learned in the context of the training to a broader set of contexts. In cognitive remediation, this process of generalization refers to the application of cognitive skills and compensatory strategies acquired in the Neuropsychological and Educational Approach to Cognitive Remediation (NEAR) sessions to circumstances and situations outside of the NEAR group. For example, a client may have practiced several memory techniques while working on Frippletration, an attention and memory exercise. These memory techniques could consist of using an organized, systematic approach and verbalizing what one sees when exposing the stimuli in the game. Evidence of generalization of these techniques would be that this individual was able to use these strategies in his home, for example, when cleaning and rearranging his belongings so that he could remember where he placed things. Another example of generalization comes from the following case example:

> M.H. is a 29-year-old woman with schizophrenia and a history of substance abuse currently in remission. She has had fairly good positive symptom control, but continues to struggle with cognitive impairment, sensitivity to noise and movement, and social isolation. She has attended cognitive remediation for several months, working on attention, sequencing, planning, and organization. It was initially difficult to match her with computer-based activities because of her sensitivities to sound and movement, but these seemed to lessen over time. She spent several weeks mastering Stocktopus, an activity that helps people to plan and sequence, and develop working memory. During a group discussion about cognition, she pronounced to another client that the computer activities are very helpful. She said, "You don't realize it at first, but then you just start using the skills in your

everyday life. Like when I need to go to the gym. Now I think about the steps, like what I need to bring and how I'm going to get there, things like that."

M.H.'s vignette presents an example of a generalized skill, metacognition, knowledge and awareness of one's own cognitive processes, as well as insight. Further, the statement was made during a bridging group. Bridging groups are an integral part of NEAR as they help to link the cognitive skills learned on computer tasks to everyday life. Bridging groups are verbal groups composed of the clients who are taking part in cognitive remediation. The content of these groups ranges from discussing the cognitive remediation software and the cognitive problems that they address to providing exercises in cognition that are not computer based. The following section provides several examples of the various types of bridging groups.

Metacognitive Groups

Metacognitive groups emphasize self-evaluation and reflection, "thinking about one's thinking," in order to enhance compensatory and adaptive approaches in real-life situations. These groups encourage people to reflect on their unique learning styles, the way they approach cognitive challenges, and the cognitive processes they use to negotiate everyday tasks

One of the first bridging groups should be a discussion about the cognitive remediation activities themselves—what do they help with? How can using these activities be helpful in everyday life? Helping clients to understand these important issues will lead to greater intrinsic motivation as well as help clients to integrate skills and strategies into their day-to-day activities. The goals of this type of group are to help clients to understand what we mean by cognition, to help them to identify their own cognitive processes, and to connect some of the computer activities to cognitive skills. This should be the first bridging group, but is one that should be returned to as clients progress in cognitive remediation and as they gain exposure to different computer programs. Reinforcing the connection between activities performed in

The Learning Center with everyday life is something that should be done often on an individual and group level.

The following dialogue is an example of how the initial bridging group on this topic might progress:

Therapist: Today we are going to step away from our computer-based activities to talk about cognition. What is cognition?

Debbie: Is it how smart you are?

Eric: I think cognition means how good your attention is.

Stanley: I had cognitive-behavioral therapy, so maybe it has to do with that.

Therapist: Those are all great ideas. First, Stan, you are right that cognition is a word used in cognitive-behavioral therapy. In that treatment cognition refers to your thoughts. In cognitive remediation it refers to your thinking skills. Eric, you were on the right track; attention is one of the skills that we refer to when we say cognition, but we also mean memory, concentration, and how we stay organized and solve problems. Cognition is not the same as how smart you are, but if you are able to remember things and solve problems, do you think you will be able to be a better learner?

Debbie: Yes!

Therapist: So good cognitive skills can help us to get smarter.

Robbie: I want to go back to school.

Therapist: That's a great goal, Robbie, and working on your cognitive skills is a great way to help you to reach that goal. So again, when we are talking about cognitive skills and cognition, we are talking about memory, attention, concentration, organization, and solving problems. Does anyone here have trouble with any of these things?

Stanley: I have trouble paying attention.

Sheila: My memory is no good. I forget stuff all the time. My mother always gets mad at me because I keep losing my bus pass.

Robbie: I don't have any problems like that.

Therapist: Robbie, even if you aren't noticing problems with your cognitive skills, because you want to go back to school, perhaps you can work on sharpening your skills. Even top athletes continue to train—as humans, we always have room to grow.

Robbie: I guess it would be helpful to learn to memorize better.

Therapist: That sounds good, Robbie. So let's talk about some of the programs we have been using so we can understand what they help us with and how they do it. Can someone mention a game you have been working on?

Sheila: Frippletration.

Stanley: Me too.

Therapist: Great. I think everyone here has tried that program at least once, right? Does someone have a guess about what cognitive skills the program makes you use?

Sheila: I think it makes me use my memory.

Therapist: That's right, Sheila; playing that game does make you use your memory. Can you describe how it does that?

Sheila: Well, you have these squares, and there is stuff behind them; you have to remember what's behind each one and make the matches.

Eric: Yeah, and sometimes you have to remember things like shapes, and sometimes it's things you hear.

Therapist: Can anyone think of a situation in real life when you have to remember something you see or something you hear?

Robbie: My friend Hector called me the other day to meet him for lunch. He told me the name of the restaurant, but I forgot the name and couldn't find it. I didn't make it, and he was annoyed.

Therapist: Thanks Robbie; that's a great example of a situation from real life where remembering what you heard was very important. Does anyone else have an example of a situation where memory was important?

Debbie: Well, I always forget to take things with me when I leave my house. Like the other day I went to the supermarket and I forgot my shopping list. I didn't know what to get. I ended up getting chips and some apples. Then I got home and saw I needed milk and some other things.

Therapist: That's a great example, Debbie. There were actually two parts in that story about remembering. One was that you forgot to take the list with you, and the second was that you could not remember items from the list without it. It sounds like working on memory and improving memory would be very helpful to many of the group members in everyday life.

Name That Cognitive Skill

Bridging groups can also include exercises where the group is presented with a scenario and is asked to brainstorm about the cognitive skills needed for the character in the scenario to be successful, the compensatory strategies that can be utilized, and the cognitive remediation exercises that can be used to bolster the needed skills. The following is an example:

> Britney went to her doctor yesterday at 11 a.m. on 45th street and 5th Avenue for a regular checkup. The doctor measured her blood pressure and weight, and gave her a physical exam. He mentioned that her blood pressure was slightly elevated and she had gained 20 pounds over the last 6 months. He told her that she should take care of herself or she would risk heart disease and diabetes. He made several suggestions. First, Britney would have to change her diet. She could make an appointment with a nutritionist or she could buy a book about a healthy, low-salt, low-fat diet. Either way, she should be careful about what she eats. The doctor also prescribed a new medicine for her blood pressure and gave her the prescription to have filled. He then asked her if she needed refills on any of her existing medications.

After reviewing the case example, you may wish to ask the group the following questions:

■ What cognitive skills did Britney need to use in order to get to her doctor's appointment?
  Possible answers include memory (I have an appointment with my doctor at 11 a.m.) and planning (scheduling a wake-up time,

making travel arrangements, identifying items to bring to the appointment, etc.).

- What skills did Britney have to use while she was in the doctor's office?
  Possible answers include attention (paying attention to what the doctor is saying), information processing (Do I have questions about what the doctor is telling me?), social skills (being assertive and asking questions, or asking the doctor to explain or repeat himself), and learning and memory (I have to remember all the things the doctor is telling me).

- What skills will Britney have to use after leaving the office to follow all of his recommendations?
  Possible answers include planning (follow-through on the many tasks the doctor gave me), problem solving (Should I call a nutritionist? How do I find one? Should I get a book instead? Where do I go?), and memory (I have to drop off a prescription).

- What can Britney do to make some of these tasks easier for herself?
  Possible answers include plan the night before the visit to have the necessary items prepared and set her alarm clock; bring a pen and paper to her appointment so she can write down what the doctor says; ask the doctor to give her written instructions and information; and call a family member, friend, or social worker for help if needed.

- What activities in The Learning Center might help Britney if she struggled with any of these tasks?
  Possible answers include Frippletration for memory; Factory Deluxe for planning and breaking down problems into steps; Stocktopus for planning and working memory; and Carmen USA for information processing, maintaining activities toward a goal, etc.

- Has anyone here had a similar experience to Britney and had some difficulty? This question helps to bridge from the abstract example to clients' own lives and experiences.

What's Happening in My Life?

As clients gain an understanding of cognition and how their cognitive skills play a part in their everyday activities, bridging groups can begin to integrate clients' own success and failure experiences in everyday life as topics of brainstorming and discussion. Successes are a source of pride, and most clients feel good sharing these positive experiences with the group. Other group members who may be struggling can gain inspiration from a successful peer. Alternatively, real-world situations in which clients had difficulty provide an opportunity for the group to identify strategies and techniques that can help the individual to be more successful the next time he is in a similar situation. This also provides an opportunity for clients to identify with each other through sharing difficulties with everyday tasks. Finally, having clients present scenarios from their own lives is a cognitive and social activity in itself for both the speaker and the listeners. Presenting a set of ideas or an experience requires forethought, planning, organization, oral presentation skills, and the ability to attend to and process questions and suggestions from the group. The group is tasked with paying attention and using active listening skills, then processing the information, analyzing the problem presented, and generating relevant commentary and/or suggestions.

Sometimes we call the group *Talk About It!* It is a content-driven, discussion group that may be used to highlight awareness of cognitive deficits. *Talk About It!* promotes support and identification, interpersonal interaction, and social skills development and is based on a recovery-oriented focus. It relies on a theme or topical discussion, such as how to follow directions, how to think before you act, or how to look for essential information. A product or self-help guide can be the result of ongoing discussions among stable group members. For example, members of one *Talk About It!* group produced a guide called *Everything You Wanted to Know About How to Improve Your Thinking Skills* with 16 helpful hints that were generated from topical discussions about cognitive functioning. It allowed the participants to identify with peers, get support, develop social skills, and to be proactive in recovery.

What's Your Learning Style?

While understanding that cognition is an important aspect in gaining insight into how one functions in the world, it is equally important to have knowledge and insight about one's learning style. Learning styles are individual preferences for taking in, processing, organizing, and learning information. They refer to the time of day one learns at his best, sensory style (the medium by which one takes in the most information), organizational style (the way in which one prefers information to be delivered), and social learning style.

Time Factors

Everyone learns best when they are well rested. Ask clients when they feel they are at their best, when they are the most sharp. Some people will report that they are "morning people" and feel best taking in new information and new challenges early in the day. They may report becoming less alert as the day progresses and have an early bedtime. Others will note a preference for learning later in the day, or even at night. Many people will never have thought about it. This conversation should get people thinking about when they are at their best. Next, begin a discussion about the maximum length of time people feel attentive. This can vary widely as well. Some clients may not have thought about this as an issue in their current lives, but will be able to think back to their attentional capacities when they were children or when in school most recently.

Sensory Style

This refers to the method by which information is communicated. Some people prefer to read information, others like to have it told to them, and still others prefer graphical information. Oftentimes, individuals learn best through some combination of the three. Discussion about mediums should get clients thinking about how they learn best. This is useful knowledge because we are all challenged to learn on a daily basis. For example, knowing you need a combination of verbal and written material is useful information when you are in a doctor's office receiving lengthy and complex instructions.

Organizational Style

How people take in complex, interrelated material is also highly individual. Some people prefer to see the big picture first, to get a global understanding of the issue. For "big picture" folks, being faced with all the details results in their getting lost in them. Conversely, others need to approach complex issues by examining all the parts or details systematically and working toward seeing the big picture. To the detail-oriented learner, trying to manage the big picture without having a careful understanding of the component parts can be simply overwhelming. Have clients discuss their preferences and style as it relates to details.

Social Learning Style

Most learning does not occur in social isolation. Usually one interacts with others—perhaps a supervisor on the job, a teacher, peers, or a family member. An individual's personality, style, and social preferences will affect how that person learns in a given situation. For example, some people need to appear competent and in charge, whereas for others it is important to be seen as useful and helpful. Some people want to learn independently, whereas others seek frequent assistance and guidance before trying something independently.

The following is an example of how a session about learning styles might progress:

Therapist: Today I want to have a group discussion about learning styles. What I mean by learning styles is that we all take in and learn information differently. For example, some people really like to read books, and others prefer to wait and learn about something from the movie. There are lots of factors that can make learning easier or more difficult for us, but it's all really personal. What works for you, Janet, may not work for you, Dave. So let's get this started and explore our learning styles.

Dave, are you a morning person or an evening person? If you have to read new information and learn it, say for work or school, would you rather do it in the morning or afternoon?

Dave: Oh! I am definitely an afternoon person.

Janet: Not me, I like mornings. I like to get up early, like 5 a.m., make coffee, and watch the early news shows.

Dave: I can't even think in the morning! It takes me until like noon until I feel like my medication has worn off.

Therapist: So Dave, what happens, then, if someone gives you things to do in the morning and you are a night person?

Dave: I won't do a very good job, I think.

Therapist: And Janet, you like the mornings, so if I asked you to read two chapters from a textbook at 10 p.m., would you be ready to answer questions for the quiz the next day?

Janet: I don't know. It would be hard to read that late. I am so tired by 10 p.m.

Therapist: So what would be a better thing to do?

Janet: Read in the morning, I guess.

Therapist: Exactly! Knowing your learning style helps you to determine when and how to set up a learning situation, like reading a book, so you have a good chance of learning and remembering something new.

Therapist: Christopher, are you someone who likes to think of many different things at once or stick with one idea?

Christopher: I don't know.

Therapist: Well, for example, if you go to the grocery store, do you follow the list or get ideas as you go along?

Cognitive Skills Building Groups

Skills building groups differ from metacognitive groups because the focus is on the remediation of specific cognitive deficits as opposed to increasing awareness about cognition. Skills building groups may teach compensatory strategies, identify adaptive mechanisms for coping with cognitive impairment, or give exercises intended to improve a specific cognitive function. Multiple examples of skills building groups are described in the sections that follow.

Current Events Group

Current events groups are a great way to practice cognitive skills as well as to incorporate social skills into cognitive remediation. This type of group has to be attempted with clients who can reliably do homework, as it involves assigning homework to read an article from a local paper, and present the information from the article to the group during the next session. While one group member is making a presentation, the other group members are tasked with listening and remembering what the presenter has discussed. Many cognitive remediation participants complain of difficulty paying attention during conversations and forgetting what was said to them. Further, difficulties with conversation initiation and maintenance, above and beyond the cognitive skills that are necessary to do so, are also often present and can be addressed with this exercise. Some clients want to improve social interactions, and talking about current events provides them with material for conversations. Additionally, newspapers are an excellent tool for this type of exercise because they are socially valued, and clients feel proud to read and present information from the newspaper. It is socially valued to be informed about current events, and the current events group helps clients to engage in the world around them, while practicing their cognitive skills.

Here's an example of how an initial current events presentation and ensuing discussion might go:

Therapist: Good morning everyone!

Group: Hi.

Therapist: As you know, today we will be reviewing articles from newspapers. One person will present an article, while the rest of us will listen. Then we will all have a chance to ask questions and discuss what we've learned. Before we start, I wanted to check in with people about why we are doing this exercise in a cognitive remediation group. What do people think?

Wendy: Because reading takes concentration.

Therapist: Good point, Wendy. That is one of the reasons. What are some others? What are some things that have to happen before you start reading an article?

John: You need to get a newspaper.

Seth: Yeah, and decide which one. I like the Daily News.

Therapist: So I think what John and Seth are saying is that deciding on which newspaper and planning how, when, and where you are going to get it are some steps that have to come first, before reading.

Seth: I actually forgot until this morning, but the coffee cart outside has the Daily News, and I bought one today. Can I read an article now?

Therapist: Well Seth, I think it would distract you from the group if you read something now, but you bring up a good point about another cognitive skill we need before we even start to read.

Seth: I don't know what you mean.

Therapist: Can anyone help Seth out?

Sasha: Seth forgot the homework.

Therapist: So what cognitive skill are we talking about then?

Sasha: Memory!

Therapist: That's right! To do this homework, and to do many tasks in our everyday lives, we need memory. In this case, it's memory to do something in the future. Can people think of other examples of things they have to do in everyday life that require remembering to do something?

Wendy: My laundry. I never remember until I am out of clothes.

Jennifer: I have to remember to see my doctor.

Therapist: Both great examples. So we see already that this current events assignment involves planning, and decisions, and memory, as well as concentration. So let's get started. How many people have prepared an article? Good. OK, does anyone want to start?
[Jennifer reports on an article from the New York Times on running indoors versus outdoors.]

Therapist: Thanks, Jennifer. That was an excellent summary of the article. Does anyone have questions about Jennifer's article?

Seth: I sometimes go for a jog around my neighborhood.

Therapist: So Seth, based on the article, do you think it's a good idea or a bad idea to run outside?

Seth: Um . . . I'm not sure . . . I don't think I was paying too much attention.

Therapist: It can be difficult to pay attention to what others are saying, and when that happens, we can miss a lot of important information. Can someone help out Seth?

Wendy: Jennifer, didn't you say that running outside can be bad for you because you can hurt yourself if the ground is uneven?

Jennifer: Yes, but you burn more calories outside than on a treadmill.

Seth: Oh, so I am burning more calories. That's a good thing.

Therapist: Good job paying attention, Seth. What's the risk of running outside that Wendy mentioned?

Seth: I could hurt myself. But don't worry Wendy, I'm really careful. I don't even run that far.

John: Can I talk about my article now?

Problem Solving Group

Another type of learning group focuses on mutual problem solving by posing real-life scenarios for group discussion. Following are several examples of problem solving groups.

Example 1

Charlie has a date tomorrow, but his apartment is a mess; he has no food or drinks in the refrigerator, he has no clean clothes left, and he's starting to panic. He told his date to meet him at his place and then he will take her to a movie. She left it up to Charlie to pick the movie. He has only a day to get everything in order, and he doesn't even know where to start. Can you help Charlie?

Sample group questions:

■ As a group, can we make a list of things that Charlie has to accomplish before tomorrow's date?
Possible answers include the following: Choose a movie theater, pick a movie, and choose a movie time; clean apartment, do laundry; buy items he might serve to his date, etc.

■ Does it matter what he does first?
This question is useful to get the group talking about prioritization, time management, and problem solving.

■ How can he be sure to get everything done?
This question is useful to get the group talking about time management, list making, and organization.

■ What's the most important thing Charlie has to do?
This question is useful to get the group talking about prioritization and time management.

■ What activities in The Learning Center could Charlie use to help strengthen his planning and organization skills?
Possible answers include the following: Carmen USA/World, Stocktopus, Fripplehouse, Factory Deluxe, Hot Dog Stand, and preparing an article for a newsletter.

Example 2

Paula has an appointment at Gotham Hospital at 12:30 with Dr. Singh. She takes the hospital address and the doctor's phone number with her. She gets to the hospital right on time, but can't seem to find the doctor's office. How can she find out how to get to the doctor's office?

Sample group questions:

- How do we solve this problem?

- Which software programs that we use here would help Paula to solve her problem? Why?

Cognitive skills needed for this problem: Memory, memory strategies, problem solving, map reading, spatial reasoning.

Example 3

Lamar just got a job stocking shelves in a supermarket. For his first assignment, his boss asks him to arrange all the canned vegetables in alphabetical order. What is the best way for Lamar to go about accomplishing this task?

Sample group questions:

- How do we solve this problem?

- Which programs in The Learning Center would give Lamar the skills to solve this problem?

Cognitive skills needed for this problem: Sequencing, spelling, problem solving, attention, time management.

Example 4

Catherine works in an office as a secretary for three people. Sometimes they all want her to do things at the same time. One wants her to make reservations at a restaurant for next Tuesday at 8 p.m. for four people, another boss wants her to make 10 photocopies of a document for tomorrow, and another boss asks her to come into his office immediately and take dictation. Catherine has difficulty remembering all of these things and is afraid she will get in trouble if she messes any of them up. How should Catherine make sure she gets everything done right?

Sample group questions:

■ How do we solve this problem?

■ What programs in The Learning Center would give Catherine the skills she needs here?

Cognitive skills needed for this problem: Memory, attention, concentration, sequencing, problem solving, organization, time management, procedural memory, spelling, processing speed.

Example 5

Homer wants to surprise his girlfriend tomorrow by baking her a birthday cake. The problem is he doesn't have a recipe or any of the ingredients. What should Homer do?

Sample group questions:

■ How do we solve this problem?

■ Where should Homer get a cake recipe from?

■ How will he remember what ingredients to get from the store?

■ What programs in The Learning Center would help Homer learn the skills he needs to solve this problem?

Cognitive skills needed for this problem: Problem solving, sequencing, memory, organization, planning, attention, arithmetic.

Newsletter Group

One example of a group task is a newsletter group. A newsletter group brings a group of individuals together to produce a common product, but allows for individual expression and assignments, and facilitates written communication skills that organize thinking. The variety of assignments allows for optimum individualization of goals based on cognitive functioning and goals for treatment. For example, some clients can work on layout, others can make a cartoon or picture, one can write a movie or software review, and another can write up an interview of someone they find interesting. Clients who can handle distal, less defined goals can simply be given the task of writing an article and taught to brainstorm what their topic will be. Clients who require more defined goals may do well to be given a choice of two or three topics and then provided with a rubric for organizing the material. There are readily available formats for newsletters that are available on the word processing programs that come with most computers.

Presenting an Argument

Another example of a group task is to work together to present a winning argument for doing something the group wants. For example, the group may want to send a persuasive letter to the administrator asking for a new computer or printer. To do this, teach them these steps to make a persuasive argument (Monroe, 1975):

1. Get attention with a strong statement of the problem. Example: "Computers have made it possible for people to work on their thinking skills."

2. Show the need by describing the problem. Example: "We are members of The Learning Center and come here to work on improving our thinking skills. However, there are not enough computers for us to work on."

3. Present a solution to the problem. Example: "We need another computer so that everyone attending The Learning Center is able to work on improving their thinking skills."

4. Visualize the benefits of the solution. Example: "If there were another computer at The Learning Center, then more people in this program could improve their thinking skills, which in turn would help them reach their treatment goals."

5. Request action. Example: "We can identify the computer that we would recommend and suggest that an order be placed."

Goals for individuals can include the ability to focus, identify the steps to reach a goal, and work together to problem solve and communicate effectively. The emphasis is on verbal communication, sequencing, organization, and planning skills. A task group such as this is useful for transfer of skills into real-world activities, like communicating a proposal to others.

Paper and Pencil Tasks

Another task-oriented group may focus on paper and pencil exercises that could be tailored to individual needs in order to remediate specific cognitive skills such as oral comprehension and visual discrimination. Tasks may place emphasis on auditory processing, attention to detail, concentration, and working memory. Although the tasks can be individually selected, and self-paced, and performed in parallel fashion, they can also be done cooperatively within teams to foster social interaction. There are numerous paper and pencil problem solving tasks available on the Web site www.puzzles.com. For example, more logic problems like the problem solving task used in the assessment (see page 66) can be downloaded and done as a group activity. Also, many of the educational software programs come with a teacher's guide that includes paper and pencil tasks to augment the software activity.

Games: "Laughing & Learning Group"

The "Laughing & Learning Group" is a popular NEAR activity. The group aim is to enhance cognition in a playful and motivating context using structured games. In addition, social skills and interpersonal problem solving are facilitated by using teams and structured interactions. Specific games can foster sustained, selective, and divided attention, working memory, and various forms of problem solving. Popular activities include telling jokes for immediate recall; card games such as SET® and Blink for working memory, reasoning, and cognitive flexibility; and Scattergories for verbal fluency, conceptualization, and categorization. Educational games and parlor activities are excellent resources for the group therapist. Task analysis that reviews the underlying cognitive demands is required, which also allows the therapist to explain to group members what the therapeutic value of the activities might be in addition to the pleasure and fun of playing.

Summary

This chapter has reviewed how to design and implement group activities for individuals with cognitive deficits. Most importantly, there has been an emphasis on the need for positive experiences in order to "broaden and build" and to structure experiences that optimally bridge thought and action in group settings. Focus on strengths as well as deficits. Offer positive reinforcement and encouragement, even in the midst of lowered expectations. Remember that individuals with cognitive dysfunction work harder and longer to accomplish the same goals. Do not look for quick solutions; good outcomes depend on severity of cognitive deficits, prior levels of functioning, current phase of recovery, and the therapeutic facilitation of goals. Place an emphasis on functional outcome. Be willing to confront cognitive dysfunction as an independent symptom cluster and specific target for treatment. Practice patience, flexibility, and creativity in executing group leadership roles. Use activities that address multiple alternate learning styles and provide instructional techniques that maximize each participant's functioning. Always be creative, and explore new group modalities that offer structure and support for those with cognitive deficits.

Chapter 10 | *Dealing With Difficult Clinical Situations*

Clients can sometimes present with behaviors that are counterproductive to learning, or that interfere with the overall goal-oriented atmosphere in The Learning Center. The vignettes presented in this chapter are not intended to fully describe any one case, but rather to highlight how to deal with some issues that commonly arise within cognitive remediation programs.

The Client Who Is Constantly in Motion

Some people have trouble sitting still. Their foot taps constantly, they fidget in their seat or, more problematically, they move the computer mouse constantly. Not only does this make it difficult for them to work on tasks, but it can also distract people working nearby.

Hypothesize and Investigate

The first step in dealing with a problem such as this is to think about why it is happening. Is the client suffering from a medication side effect? Is the client's movement a manifestation of anxiety or attention-deficit hyperactivity disorder (ADHD)? Or is this simply the client's style? Looking at the client's history and talking to other members of the team can be helpful in establishing whether the restlessness is apparent in other settings as well. If it is, then consider the issue of medication side effects or ADHD and ask the client's psychiatrist for her opinion. Assuming it is not a symptom best addressed by medication changes, this is something that can be addressed in the cognitive remediation sessions.

Encourage Awareness

In a nonjudgmental, friendly manner say to the client, *"I notice that you* . . . (keep your legs moving; keep moving the mouse; move a lot). *"* Determine whether the client is aware of this, and ask her to explain it. Sometimes your statement serves to plant the seeds of awareness. Sometimes the client will say something like, *"I've always been like that,"* or *"I get anxious."* If the client demonstrates little or no awareness, you will need to keep making one comment per session for several sessions until she starts to show recognition of her movements.

Consider the Adaptive Effects of the Movements

Make a simple statement to the client such as, *"Foot tapping can sometimes help a person feel more comfortable."* Allow the client to reflect on how the movement helps her in some way. This is important to do so the person feels understood. It also prepares the client for dealing with the loss she might experience when she eventually tries to change the habit.

Consider the Disruptive Effects of the Movements, and Offer an Alternative

This must be delicately done—and at a time when the person can readily see that the moving is interfering with her ability to work on the computer. Therefore, this step must be taken once the person is engaged in an activity. Say something like this: *"When you move the mouse all the time, it can make it hard to play this game. How about you try to move your leg or tap your foot, and practice keeping this arm and hand still?"* Suggest that the movements be confined to one limb, a foot or lower leg. This isolates and contains the movement so that it will be less disruptive.

Suggest Periodic Stretches

Some people do well to get up and stretch every 30 min. Say something like this: *"How about you give yourself a break and get up and stretch? It can be hard to sit for long periods, and we are often better able to concentrate after a little exercise."*

The Client With Poor Mouse Control

Many clients, particularly adults who have not had much experience using computers, find it difficult to smoothly move the mouse. They jerk and shake it, cannot move it to a designated target, and have difficulty making it stay in one place. The following exercises can be used to help the person develop better mouse control.

1. You or the client may type her name and the names of people she knows in a line repetitively until there are four lines, and then make the lines have fonts of different sizes, ranging from 18 to 14. Once this is done, have the client point the mouse and click and delete all the letter A's, and then all the letter B's, and so on, until most of the letters have been deleted.

2. Look for a software program that requires basic mouse control, such as Quick Change from Math Arena™, and then turn the timer off so that the client can focus on mouse control while still developing attention and problem solving strategies.

3. Consider using a prosthetic device. Sometimes it helps to put a wrist weight on the arm that controls the mouse. This provides a visual and proprioceptive cue that reminds the person to move smoothly. It can also help stabilize the wrist in people with movement disorders.

The Client Who Is Perpetually Late or Absent

The perpetually late or frequently absent client represents a particular challenge to the cognitive rehabilitation specialist. To address this issue with the client, the CRS must consider the following issues: (1) limit setting, (2) assigning value to participation in The Learning Center, (3) involving the entire treatment team, and (4) cultural/social factors.

Limit Setting

The perpetually late client may not know what is expected of her at The Learning Center. Although the rules may have been delineated during an initial interview, the client may have forgotten them or may not have taken them seriously. The first reminder to the client should include the rationale for timely attendance. That is, it should be explained that the client will benefit only from consistent attendance to full sessions. Sporadic attendance and perpetually late arrivals will not afford the necessary exposure to and practice with the materials. It may be useful to describe this in alternate terms to make certain the client understands the point. One metaphor that may be useful is exercise. Explain to the client that working on thinking skills is like trying to build one's muscles or lose weight. Going to the gym once a week for 20 min is not going to achieve the desired results. It is the same idea at The Learning Center. The client will not be able to achieve her goals without appearing for the whole session as scheduled.

The second reminder should follow if the client continues to arrive late for sessions. Ask the client if she remembers the first time you talked about this problem. Then, ask the client what factors are making it difficult to be punctual, and problem solve with her to deal with these factors. Does she need an alarm clock, is she giving herself enough time in the morning, is it a function of the transportation schedule, or are medications adjusted properly so she is alert in the morning? Finally, if it is clear that the lateness is habit and not cognitively or circumstance based, set limits with the client. Let the client know that she will not be allowed to join mid-session. If the client is not present within 10 min of the start of a session, she will lose that session and have to make a more concerted effort to come on time to the next group.

If the client still cannot make it to sessions on time, offer a third and final warning. Tell the client that if she is late to the next session, she will be put on "visitor status" until she can demonstrate that she can be punctual. If the client does not respond to this final warning and indeed comes late to another session, sit down with her and explain why the program does not seem to be appropriate at this time. Tell the client that she will be welcomed back in the future when it is determined that she can attend regularly and on time. In the meantime, she will be on visitor status, which means that she is not officially part of the group but can visit and, if there are free computers, can work on an activity. Because the group will comprise people who can make a commitment to attend, it is likely that when clients on visitor status drop by, they will see a room full of people at work at the computers. If they liked being in The Learning Center, and the CRS handled their lateness in a non-judgmental way, seeing peers at work will give them some incentive to improve or change. Some clients will ultimately prove to be appropriate referrals and will demonstrate a vastly improved attendance record.

Assigning Value to The Learning Center

Clients will take a more serious attitude toward attendance and punctuality if they value the activities performed at The Learning Center. This may occur naturally as they become more adept at operating the computer and software and feel more skilled at the tasks. Others value The Learning Center when they understand how the skills they are learning may be useful in attaining employment or otherwise meeting their recovery goals. For still others, it might require giving them a position of perceived importance within The Learning Center, such as attendance monitor, software expert, newsletter editor, peer advisor, etc. Being given a position provides an additional sense of belonging and importance and usually results in improved attendance. Similarly, matching clients with peers, with whom they are assigned to work, may improve attendance by creating a sense of collaboration.

Involving the Entire Treatment Team

The client with poor attendance and poor punctuality to The Learning Center likely has the same issues with other appointments (e.g., psychiatrist, social worker, job interview) on her schedule. The client's team may or may not be aware of this pattern of behavior. Making them aware of this issue is extremely important. If the client is missing other appointments, she may not have sufficient medication, may not be medically stable, or may be sabotaging potential employment. If other team members are aware of the problem, the team meeting can provide a forum to discuss underlying reasons for the client's behavior as well as possible interventions. Further, having other members of the client's team reinforce to the client the importance of punctuality and attendance to their sessions in The Learning Center can only increase the chance of your client improving those behaviors.

Cultural/Social Factors

Whenever attempting to understand a client's behavior and make the appropriate behavioral interventions, it is important to consider if there are cultural factors at work. Whereas Western culture places great value and emphasis on punctuality, some other cultures may not share that custom. The concept of a dedicated time set aside for a specific purpose may be a foreign notion, which may have to be explained and reiterated. Further, many clients of lower socioeconomic status have experienced a lifetime of long waits in emergency rooms and clinic waiting areas; they themselves have not been given much respect in terms of timely service. In other words, others may have set a bad example of the importance of punctuality, and the client may only be displaying learned behaviors.

The Client Who Needs Constant Feedback

Another type of difficult client is the one who needs constant feedback. A needy client can be difficult to work with for two reasons: (1) The CRS may begin to resent the need for constant affirmation and feedback, and (2) The CRS working with a group of people may find most of her time consumed with the client who requires constant feedback and attention, and may not be able to attend to the needs of the other clients in the room. The implications and solutions to each of these problems are outlined in the sections that follow.

The CRS's Reaction

One of the major challenges of working with the needy client is the cumulative effect of the client's constant needs on the CRS. Similar to the concept of countertransference in the context of the therapeutic relationship, the CRS may unconsciously become affected by the behavior of the client. In this case, there is a danger that the CRS may begin to resent the client or dread the client's appointment times. Without being cognizant of this process, the CRS may begin to treat the needy client differently, or become short-tempered or even sarcastic. By becoming aware of the dangers of working with this type of client, the CRS can monitor her own reactions and avoid treating the client in a negative manner.

If the CRS finds herself reacting negatively toward the needy client, she can use that reaction to guide interventions and improve her understanding of the client and how the client interacts with others. If the client is having this effect on the CRS, it is likely that she has the same effect on friends, family, and employers. One can immediately understand how this client may have difficulty in a variety of situations (work/home) as a result of her constant need for feedback, which places potentially overwhelming demands on others' time and attention. In recognizing this, the CRS has identified one possible pitfall, or stumbling block, that may interfere with the client's ability to achieve her goals. This then becomes as important a target of the cognitive remediation as the cognitive deficits, because without self-confidence how will the client be able to use her cognitive skills? First, the CRS must realize that a client who needs constant feedback is lacking in self-esteem and ego strength, resulting in a constant need for praise and validation from external sources. An individual such as this is not capable of recognizing her own successes and feeling proud of herself. This person has become accustomed to placing value on only those achievements that garner external recognition. The CRS must wean the client slowly from her dependence on this external affirmation and have her learn to recognize, value, and feel pride in her own accomplishments.

Moving a client from a position of dependence to one of self-sufficiency and pride is a slow process. If the CRS becomes too withholding, too quickly, the client will not feel successful in her activities, may lose interest in attending The Learning Center, and may begin to come to sessions late, or begin to miss sessions altogether. Rather, the CRS must initially provide the praise and support the client needs. It is important to first establish The Learning Center as a place where the client experiences success, praise, achievement, and accomplishment. As indicated in previous chapters, establishing a strong relationship with the client and creating a comfortable environment is the key to establishing a positive learning environment. Only after the client is comfortable and has had consistent experiences of success can she begin to tolerate receiving less external praise. The CRS can begin this process by bringing the problem into the client's awareness with statements like, *"It seems like often you can't tell if you have done a good job,"* or *"You really like me to see your work on this task!"* In an effort to get the client to begin to recognize her own achievements, the CRS may ask the client to explain her progress in a given task prior to the client requesting feedback or praise. For example, if the client is engaged in Fripplehouse, the CRS might ask her to explain how she approached the task and whether she thinks that was a good strategy. Help the client learn to accurately rate her own effort and level of skill with statements like *"I would like to hear about how you did this. Tell me, how did you deal with it when you had to . . . ? And did that work? When did you know you were on to a good strategy? It must feel good to have figured that out!"* These statements emphasize the process of learning and place the CRS in the position of showing interest in the learning style and not the performance outcome. As the client gains self-confidence and learns to recognize her own progress, she will begin to require less praise and will develop a stronger sense of self and self-esteem. That is not to say that there is no room for praise from the CRS. Everyone appreciates recognition, but it is even more valuable when it comes less frequently and confirms self-evaluation rather than when it is the sole source of evaluation.

The Needy Client Is Taking Time Away From the Other Clients

If the needy client shares The Learning Center with other clients, the CRS may find it difficult to give the other clients the time and attention they need. This may add to the negative countertransference discussed previously, and may also cause other clients to have a negative experience in The Learning Center as their needs may go unmet. It is the CRS's responsibility to achieve a balance in The Learning Center. In this case, the CRS may have to let the needy client know that although her needs are very important to the CRS, she cannot devote all her time to meeting them, saying something like *"I can see that you are doing some very good work over there, but right now I have to help* [another client] *with a problem she is having."* It is important for the needy client to recognize that others in the room have needs that are as important as her own; the CRS may have to reinforce this concept repeatedly as the client may initially have difficulty seeing past her own needs. It can be helpful to discuss nonverbal signals that the CRS and client can use so that there is not a constant calling out of demands, which might distract others in the group. The CRS can say, *"I am not always able to come over to you right when you want me, but I do often look around the room, even when I am working with someone else. So if you would like me to come over, look at me and give a thumbs-up, and I will do the same back to indicate that I see you and will come over as soon as possible."* This type of intervention shapes the demanding behavior to be less disruptive, and often the client will happily go back to work once she sees that the CRS has responded to her.

The Client Who Only Wants to Work on One Activity

Some clients happily and regularly attend The Learning Center but only want to work on one activity. Day after day they arrive, take out their folder and the same software program, and sit the whole session working on one activity. When the CRS shows them a new activity, they listen politely and immediately go back to their favorite. It is of course positive that they are so engaged, but the CRS has to consider whether this exclusive focus on one activity is therapeutic. Generally speaking, if the client is engaged in a higher-level problem solving activity like Carmen, Hot Dog Stand, or Zoombinis, it is therapeutic, because it can easily take a whole session to complete a task, the task challenges multiple cognitive skills, and it is positive to see clients aspiring to higher levels. As long as the clients are working productively, it can be quite rewarding for them to advance in the activity. However, if the CRS believes they have plateaued at a level of difficulty, it is advisable to ask them to work on a different activity. The CRS might say, *"You really like working on Carmen! I noticed you have been running out of time on the cases. It will help you to move ahead in Carmen if you work on your processing speed. I would like you to work on Combo Cubes for a while to help you think quickly. Let me show you (again) how it works."*

Not infrequently, clients, especially those who are anxious or have very low premorbid IQ, will want to work on a simple repetitive program like Frippeltration for the whole session. In general, it is not therapeutic for clients to work on the simple activities with proximal goals for more than 25 min. Unless they practice their skills in multiple contexts, it is unlikely that the gains they make will generalize to functional activities of daily living. Thus, it is important for the clinician to provide structure and guidance to these clients. Even though the Neuropsychological Educational Approach to Cognitive Remediation (NEAR) advocates giving as much learner control as possible, this should not be done at the cost of therapeutic gain. Therefore the clinician may need to assert some control over the choice of activities by saying, *"I would like you to work on two activities each session. Which two of the activities on this list do you want to work on? OK, start with this one* (the new one*), and then after 25 minutes change back to* (the old one)." One of the goals on the treatment plan should then be to increase cognitive flexibility as demonstrated by taking initiative to work on several activities in one session. If the cognitive rigidity is a reflection of anxiety, then the client should start to show more exploratory behavior once they feel confident and secure. Sometimes it can take a long time to help the rigid client become more flexible in her approach to learning.

Chapter 11 *Program Evaluation*

Program evaluation is essential to the stability and health of a program. It serves the dual purpose of monitoring performance and making others aware of the program activities. It allows supervisors and administrators to have a snapshot view of the activities of the cognitive rehabilitation specialist (CRS) and the program at large. It also allows for identification of areas that need improvement. The rationale for doing program evaluation is as follows:

1. To look at how the program is being utilized.

2. To maximize the effectiveness of the services provided.

3. To assess and improve the quality of clinical service.

4. To provide information about the functioning of the program to others.

Assessing Program Utilization

Utilization studies help to better manage the limited resources of The Learning Center so that services reach a greater number of clients. The studies should indicate patterns of utilization, including such information as the number of clients enrolled and the number of clients actually coming to sessions. If, for example, it is noted that people are not coming to scheduled sessions, then the CRS's time is not being used effectively. The CRS is waiting to work with people who are not showing up, and other patients are not getting an opportunity to attend The Learning Center. To assess utilization, use the blank Utilization Report form provided in the appendix on a quarterly basis. A sample completed form is shown in Figure 11.1.

Quarterly Utilization Report

Dates: January, February, March, 2000

Status: _____First quarter of program __X__ Continuing program

Enrollment at start of quarter: __12__

I.   Number of new clients referred: __7__

2.   Number of clients interviewed/assessed: __7__
     Follow-up rate: (#2/#1 × 100) = __100 %__

3.   Number of clients accepted into the program: __6__
     Acceptance rate: (#3/#2 × 100) = __85.7 %__

4.   Number of appointments scheduled
     a.   Total this quarter: __257__
     b.   Weekly average: __21.4__

5.   Number of appointments missed/cancelled
     a.   Total this quarter: __60__
     b.   Weekly average: __5__

6.   Utilization rates
     a.   Quarterly utilization (#4a–#5a/#4a × 100) = __76.6 %__
     b.   Weekly utilization (#4b–#5b/#4b × 100) = __76.6 %__

7.   Number of clients enrolled at end of quarter: __14__

8.   Total number of discharges this quarter: __4__
     Explanation for client discharges:

     ▪ Change in schedule (e.g., day of week, program emphasis): __1__
     ▪ Discharge from program (e.g., hospitalization, graduation): __2__
     ▪ Lack of commitment to treatment program (e.g., unexplained, frequent absences): __1__
     ▪ Clinical decision (e.g., inappropriate referral, lack of readiness to work toward goal): __0__
     ▪ Other: _____

Findings:

Utilization improved slightly. Decrease in number of absences from previous quarter.

Figure 11.1

Example of completed Quarterly Utilization Report.

Assessing utilization allows for examination of the following aspects of the program.

Number of New Clients Referred

This should be greatest when a program first starts and then should level off once the program is running. For example, in a program serving 20 clients, 6 new clients may be referred every quarter. If there is a drop in referrals, it is important to find out why. Perhaps the communication between The Learning Center and rehabilitation program staff needs to be improved. Perhaps the overall rehabilitation program is experiencing a drop in referrals. If there are too many referrals, then it is important to ensure that referrals are being dealt with expediently.

Number of Clients Interviewed/Assessed

This number allows assessment of whether referrals are in fact being processed. If referred people are not coming for intake, then that should be investigated. Ask whether this is a result of a scheduling problem or if referred clients are not pursuing intake. Identify the problem, and then take steps to fix it.

Number of Clients Accepted Into Program

This number gives an indication of the appropriateness of the referrals. If there is a discrepancy between the number referred and the number accepted, then it may be necessary to review and change the referral and intake procedures.

Number of Appointments Scheduled

This number indicates time allotted for patient care.

Number of Appointments Missed/Canceled

Those times when the client did not show up for the appointment or appointments were canceled are indicated here. It is wise to differentiate between the "no shows" and the cancellations because these indicate different clinical situations. The utilization rate indicates the percentage of scheduled sessions that are attended. If it is a low number, then steps must be taken to improve utilization. Utilization is rarely above 85%; there will always be cancellations because people have medical appointments or transportation issues or get sick. Because it is important to make efficient use of the CRS's time, scheduling extra clients or identifying and helping change the behavior of people who consistently cancel can increase utilization.

Number of Clients Enrolled

This number indicates how many people the program is serving.

Number of Discharges

The rate of discharge and reasons of discharge are presented here.

Other utilization studies can focus on the type of patients that use the service. What is the average age, education, and work history? Who are the clinicians/services that typically refer? What is the ratio of females to males? What is the primary language of the clients, and what is the ethnicity? Understanding the characteristics of the population served will assist program development.

Assessing Program Quality

The intent of the performance studies is to see if the program is effectively meeting its goals. Are the cognitive skills improving? Are clients gaining self-confidence in their ability to learn? Are clients feeling positively about this learning experience, and learning experiences in general? Are clients better able to function in treatment programs, in vocational settings, and in mainstream educational settings? In order to answer these questions, some outcome measures must be developed or designated, and then implemented at regular intervals. It is important to differentiate between subjective and objective measures of outcome. Subjective measures capture opinions, whereas objective measures compare performance to a standard. Both are valuable.

Are Cognitive Skills Improving?

To assess this, measures of cognitive ability must be taken before treatment and again after a designated time or number of sessions. Retesting is often done after 26 sessions or a designated time period like 4 months, but that is only a guideline. When choosing tests, it is important to find those that assess the skills that have been targeted by treatment.

Is Self-Confidence Improving?

There are measures of self-esteem and self efficacy available. It is important to differentiate between self-confidence in the learning situation versus other situations in life. NEAR directly targets self-esteem about learning; if there is improvement in other areas that would be a generalization of effect.

Do Clients Feel Positive About Their Experience in The Learning Center?

This question is typically answered with some sort of satisfaction survey (see appendix for sample client satisfaction questionnaires). It is useful to look at satisfaction with various aspects of the service. For example, do they feel they are seen as much as they would like, do they like working on the computers, and do they think they are being helped?

Is the Experience in The Learning Center Helping Clients Function in Other Areas of Life?

To answer this question, a combination of subjective and objective ratings can be used. Ratings of functional ability can be made by asking for the perceptions of supervisors, caseworkers, and relatives, as well as the client. Numbers of clients who go on to job training, gainful employment, or mainstream education can be obtained. The assessments should reflect the goals of the client. For example, if the goal was to return to school, then success would be measured by attainment of that goal.

Summary

When program assessment is done, the results should be analyzed and critically examined to see how the program can be improved. If clients are reporting dissatisfaction, that will need to be investigated. If cognitive skills are not improving, different techniques may need to be tried. It is not easy to measure outcome because it can be difficult to capture change with a rating scale or test. It is therefore also important to be sure that the assessments are measuring the right thing. At its best, program assessment enables the continued improvement of services, and it is therefore an important aspect of the ongoing functioning of a Learning Center.

Appendix

Referral Form

SECTION I: REFERRED CLIENT INFORMATION

Name: _____ Age: _____

Address: _____ DOB: _____

_____

Years of education: _____ Phone: _____

Diagnosis: _____

Goals: Vocational _____ Educational _____ Socialization _____

Independent living skills _____

SECTION II: REFERRAL INFORMATION

Referred by:

Agency: _____ Referral date: _____

Contact name: _____ Phone: _____

Reason(s) for referral:

   Check all that apply.

Primary: The client needs assistance with the following:

_____ Paying attention   _____ Planning skills
_____ Remembering   _____ Thinking through problems
_____ Being organized   _____ Processing information more quickly

Secondary: The client needs assistance with the following:

_____ Self-confidence   _____ Time management
_____ Ability to work with others   _____ Initiation and persistence in
                                               goal-directed activities

Additional information and/or comments:

SECTION III: COGNITIVE APPRAISAL

Please rate the referred client on the following possible areas of cognitive difficulty according to the scale below (0–5). Use your observation of the client as they function in both group and individual interactions.

Scale:

0 = Never	3 = Frequently
1 = Rarely	4 = Most of the time
2 = Occasionally	5 = Always

1. The client has trouble paying attention to conversations.   0   1   2   3   4   5

2. The client has trouble sustaining concentration in meetings.   0   1   2   3   4   5

3. The client has difficulty with memory.   0   1   2   3   4   5

4. The client has trouble finishing tasks once started.   0   1   2   3   4   5

5. The client has difficulty starting tasks.   0   1   2   3   4   5

6. The client has difficulty organizing tasks and projects.   0   1   2   3   4   5

7. The client has trouble reasoning and solving problems.   0   1   2   3   4   5

Please rank the following list of four major potential problem areas as indicated for the client in order of:

1 = the greatest problem

2 = the next greatest problem

3 = the third greatest problem

4 = the last greatest problem

_____Attention and concentration

_____Memory

_____Being organized

_____Reasoning and problem solving

Computer Task Analysis Form

Name of software program:

_____

Description of activity:

_____

_____

_____

Reading level required:

_____

Other prerequisite skills needed:

_____

_____

_____

Cognitive deficits that can be addressed:

_____

_____

_____

Goal properties:

_____

_____

_____

Computer Task Analysis Form *continued*

Adaptability of task:

Multimedia experience:

Mediation by therapist:

Overall strengths and weaknesses:

Software program name/manufacturer:

1. Cognitive deficits targeted by the software:

2. Required knowledge base

    Domain-specific knowledge:

    Reading level:

3. Working memory/attention requirements:

4. Motivation

    Intrinsic:

    Extrinsic:

5. Depth of engagement:

6. Opportunities for self-perceived competence

    Feedback provided:

    Experience of success:

7. Multisensory presentation

    Level of stimulation:

8. Contextualization

    Fantasy or real-life simulation:

    Single, multiple contexts:

    Relevance to daily life:

9. Learner controls/choice

    Difficulty levels:

    Competitive versus cooperative:

    Other:

10. Opportunities for practice

    With different cues/context:

    Within/between difficulty levels:

11. Personalization:

Assessment and Treatment Plan for Cognitive Remediation

Name: _____ Age: _____

Address: _____ DOB: _____

_____ TEL# _____

Part I: Summary of Educational Experiences

Highest grade completed: _____

Favorite subject(s) in school: _____

Worst subject(s) in school: _____

List any learning disabilities and how they are manifested:

_____

_____

_____

Enrollment in any special classes; when and where:

_____

_____

_____

Learning experience/history:

_____

_____

_____

Learning style:

_____ Auditory   _____ Visual   _____ Multisensory

_____ Independent   _____ Dependent

_____ Sitting   _____ Moving

_____ Morning   _____ Afternoon   _____ Evening

Additional information regarding learning style:

_____

_____

Familiarity with computers (check one)

_____ Very familiar   _____ Some familiarity   _____ No familiarity

continued

Part II: Summary of Work Experiences

Present position:

Where: _____

For how long: _____

Position held: _____

Number of hours worked: _____

Describe work history (positions held, successes and problems in the workplace):

_____

_____

_____

_____

Areas of concern:

_____Starting tasks   _____ Finishing tasks

_____Following directions   _____ Punctuality

_____Attendance   _____ Organization

_____Ability to work independently _____ Social: getting along with coworkers and

_____ Other   supervisors

Vocational goals:

_____

_____

_____

_____

Part III: Information Assessment

Cognitive skills assessment (from client and referral): What are the client's primary areas of weakness?

_____ Paying attention   _____ Planning skills   _____ Remembering

_____ Being organized   _____ Logic and reasoning _____ Time management

_____ Sustained concentration_____ Speed of information processing

_____ Other

Part IV: Cognitive Functions and Targeted Goals

Primary goal of program:

_____ Vocational   _____ Social

_____ Educational   _____ Living

Cognitive functions to target   Educational software

_____ Attention   Software: _____

        _____

_____ Problem solving   Software: _____

        _____

_____ Memory   Software: _____

        _____

_____ Processing speed   Software: _____

        _____

Leaning style:

Increase initiation

Intervention: _____

Increase engagement

Intervention: _____

Increase independence

Intervention: _____

Schedules session (dates and times):

_____

_____

Completed by: _____   Date: _____

Software I have learned to use Activity/disk name	What skills have I practiced?*
1.	
2.	
3.	
4.	
5.	
6.	
7.	
8.	
9.	
10.	

For example:

*problem solving   *concentration
*processing speed   *planning   *multitasking
*reasoning and logic   *attention   *organization
*quick responses   *working memory   *memory

Individual Session Log

Name: _____

Session #	Date	Software Activity disk	Level	Computer
See first row for an example				
1	04/04/09	Frippletration Thinkin' Things Collection 2	G	2

Quarterly Utilization Report

Dates: _____ to _____

Status: _____First quarter of program _____ Continuing program

Enrollment at start of quarter: _____

1. Number of new clients referred: _____

2. Number of clients interviewed/assessed: _____
   Follow-up rate: (#2/#1 × 100) = _____%

3. Number of clients accepted into the program: _____
   Acceptance rate: (#3/#2 × 100) = _____%

4. Number of appointments scheduled
   a. Total this quarter: _____
   b. Weekly average: _____

5. Number of appointments missed/cancelled
   a. Total this quarter: _____
   b. Weekly average: _____

6. Utilization rates
   a. Quarterly utilization (#4a-#5a/#4a × 100) = _____%
   b. Weekly utilization (#4b-#5b/#4b × 100) = _____%

7. Number of clients enrolled at end of quarter: _____

8. Total number of discharges this quarter: _____
   Explanation for client discharges:

   ■ Change in schedule (e.g., day of week, program emphasis): _____
   ■ Discharge from program (e.g., hospitalization, graduation): _____
   ■ Lack of commitment to treatment program (e.g., unexplained, frequent absences): _____
   ■ Clinical decision (e.g., inappropriate referral, lack of readiness to work toward goal): _____
   ■ Other: _____ ■

Findings: _____

_____

_____

_____

_____

_____

Client Satisfaction Questionnaire

Please help us improve our Learning Center program by answering some questions. We are interested in your honest opinion, whether it is positive or negative. Please answer all of the questions. Thank you.

Circle your answer

How would you rate your experience attending The Learning Center?

> 4—Excellent
>
> 3—Good
>
> 2—Fair
>
> 1—Poor

If another client at this program said they had problems with memory or attention and asked you where to get some help, would you recommend The Learning Center to him or her?

> 4—Yes, definitely
>
> 3—Yes, I think so
>
> 2—No, I don't think so
>
> 1—No, definitely not

Has attending The Learning Center helped you deal more effectively with your problems (e.g., at school or work or home or friends)?

> 4—Yes, it helped a great deal
>
> 3—Yes, it helped somewhat
>
> 2—No, it really didn't help
>
> 1—No, it seemed to make things worse

Additional feedback

Comments on your experience:

_____

_____

_____

_____

_____

Suggestions for improvement of The Learning Center:

_____

_____

_____

_____

_____

Client Questionnaire

Reactions to working in The Learning Center

1. On a scale of 1 to 10, how much did you enjoy working on the computer-based exercises at
    The Learning Center?

1	2	3	4	5	6	7	8	9	10
Not				So-so					Very
at all									much

2. On a scale from 1 to 10, how much did you like participating in the verbal groups at The
    Learning Center?

1	2	3	4	5	6	7	8	9	10
Not				So-so					Very
at all									much

3. On a scale from 1 to 10, how much would you like to continue to attend The Learning
    Center?

1	2	3	4	5	6	7	8	9	10
Not				So-so					Very
at all									much

4. In your own words, can you describe your experience at The Learning Center and how it
    relates to your goals?

    _____

    _____

    _____

    _____

References

Anthony, W. A., Cohen, M. R., Farkas, M. D., & Gagne, C. (2002). *Psychiatric Rehabilitation* (2nd ed.). Boston, MA: Boston University, Center for Psychiatric Rehabilitation.

Bark, N., Revheim, N., Huq, F., Khalderov, V., Ganz, Z. W., Medalia, A. (2003). The impact of cognitive remediation on psychiatric symptoms of schizophrenia. *Schizophrenia Research, 63*, 229–235.

Bitter, G. G., Camuse, R. A., & Durbin, V. L. (1993). *Using a microcomputer in the classroom*. Boston, MA: Allyn & Bacon.

Bowie, C. R., Leung, W. W., Reichenberg, A., McClure, M. M., Patterson, T. L., Heaton, R. K., et al. (2008). Predicting schizophrenia patients' real-world behavior with specific neuropsychological and functional capacity measures. *Biological Psychiatry, 63*(5), 505–511.

Choi, J., & Medalia, A. (2005). Factors associated with a positive response to cognitive remediation in a community psychiatric sample. *Psychiatric Services, 56*, 602–604.

Cordova, D. I., & Lepper, M. R. (1996). Intrinsic motivation and the process of learning: Beneficial effects of contextualization, personalization, and choice. *Journal of Educational Psychology, 88*(4), 715–730.

Cornblatt, B., Obuchowski, M., Schnur, D. B., & O'Brien, J. D. (1997). Attention and clinical symptoms in schizophrenia. *Psychiatric Quarterly, 68*(4), 343–359.

Dweck, C. S. (1985). Intrinsic motivation, perceived control, and self-evaluation maintenance: An achievement goal analysis. In R. Ames & C. Ames (Eds.), *Research on motivation in education* (Vol. II). New York: Academic Press.

Glahn, D. C., Bearden, C. E., Barguil, M., Barrett, J., Reichenberg, A., Bowden, C. L., et al. (2007). The neurocognitive signature of psychotic bipolar disorder. *Biological Psychiatry, 62*(8), 910–916.

Gold, J. M., & Harvey, P. D. (1993). Cognitive deficits in schizophrenia. *Psychiatric Clinics of North America, 16*(2), 295–312.

Green, M. F. (1996). What are the functional consequences of neurocognitive deficits in schizophrenia? *American Journal of Psychiatry, 153*, 321–330.

Green, M. F., Kern, R. S., Braff, D. L., & Mintz, J. (2000). Neurocognitive deficits and functional outcome in schizophrenia: are we measuring the "right stuff"? *Schizophrenia Bulletin, 26*(1), 119–136.

Hannafin, M. P., & Peck, K. L. (1998). *The design, development and evaluation of instructional software*. New York: MacMillan Publishing Company.

Hodge, M. A. R., Siciliano, D., Withey, P., Moss, B., Moore, G., Judd, G., et al. (2008). A randomized controlled trial of cognitive remediation in schizophrenia. *Schizophrenia Bulletin*, doi:10.1093/ schbul/sbn102.

Keefe, R. S., Bilder, R. M., Davis, S. M., Harvey, P. D., Palmer, B. W., Gold, J. M., et al. (2007) Neurocognitive effects of antipsychotic medications in patients with chronic schizophrenia in the CATIE Trial. *Archives of General Psychiatry, June 64*(6), 633–647.

Lieber, J., & Semmel, M. I. (1985). Effectiveness of Computer Application to Instruction with Mildly Handicapped Learners: A Review. *Remedial and Special Education (RASE), 6*(5), 5–12.

McGurk, S. R., & Meltzer, H. Y. (2000). The role of cognition in vocational functioning in schizophrenia. *Shizophrenia Research, 45*(3), 175–184.

Medalia, A., Aluma, M., Tyron, W., & Merriam, A. (1998). The effectiveness of attention training in schizophrenics. *Schizophrenia Bulletin, 24*, 147–152.

Medalia, A., Dorn, H., & Watras-Gans, S. (2000). Treating problem-solving deficits on an acute psychiatric inpatient unit. *Psychiatric research, 97*, 79–88.

Medalia, A., & Freilich, B. (2008). The NEAR Model: Practice principles and outcome studies. *American Journal of Psychiatric Rehabilitation, 11*(2), 123–143.

Medalia, A., Herlands, T., & Baginsky, C. (2003). Cognitive remediation in the supportive housing setting. *Psychiatric Services, 54*, 1219–1220.

Medalia, A., Revheim, N., & Casey, M. (2000). Remediation of memory disorders in schizophrenia. *Psychological Medicine, 30*, 1451–1459.

Medalia, A., Revheim, N., & Casey, M. (2001). The remediation of problem solving skills in schizophrenia. *Schizophrenia Bulletin, 27*(2), 259–267.

Medalia, A., Revheim, N., & Casey, M. (2002). The remedian of problem solving skills in schizophrenia: Evidence of a persistent effect. *Schizophrenia Research, 57*, 165–171.

Medalia, A., & Richardson, R. (2005). What predicts a good response to cognitive remediation interventions? *Schizophrenia Bulletin, 31*(4), 942–53.

Monroe, A. H. (1975). The motivated sequence. In B. E. Gronbeck, K. German, D. Ehninger, & A. H. Monroe (Eds.), *Principles of Speech Communication* (7th Brief ed., pp. 241–257). New York: Addison-Wesley Educational Publishers, Inc.

Revheim, N., Kamnitzer, D., Casey, M., & Medalia, A. (2001). Implementation of a cognitive rehabilitation program in an IPRT Setting. *Psychiatric Rehabilitation Skills, 5*, 403–425.

Rogers, C. R. (1967/1989). 'The interpersonal relationship in the facilitation of learning.' In H. Kirschenbaum & V. L. Henderson (Eds.), *The Carl Rogers Reader* (pp. 304–323). Houghton Mifflin.

Rogers, C. R. (1951). *Client-centered therapy: Its current practice, implications and theory.* Boston, MA: Houghton-Mifflin.

Ryan, R. M., & Deci, E. L. (2000). Self-determination theory and the facilitation of intrinsic motivation, social development, and well-being. *American Psychologist, 55*(1), 68–78.

Schunk, D. H., Pintrich, P. R., & Meece, J. (2007). *Motivation in education: Theory, research, and applications* (3rd ed.). New Jersey: Prentice Hall.

Silverstein, S. (2000). Psychiatric rehabilitation of schizophrenia: Unresolved issues, current trends, and future directions. *Applied and Preventative Psychiatry, 9*, 227–248.

Spaulding, W. D., Flemming, S. K., Reed, D., Sullivan, M., Storzbach, D., & Lam, M. (1999) Cognitive functioning in schizophrenia: Implications for psychiatric rehabilitation. *Schizophrenia Bulletin, 25*, 275–289.

Velligan, D. I., Bow-Thomas, C. C., Mahurin, R. K., Miller, A. L., & Halgunseth, L. D. (2000). Do specific neurocognitive deficits predict specific domains of community function in schizoprehnia? *The Journal of Nervous and Mental Disease, 188*(8), 518–524.

About the Authors

Alice Medalia, PhD, is Professor of Clinical Psychiatry (in Psychology) and Director of Psychiatric Rehabilitation at Columbia University College of Physicians and Surgeons. She has been working in the area of cognitive remediation for many years and is recognized as an international leader in the field. She lectures and consults to agencies worldwide and conducts training workshops for clinicians who want to learn how to provide cognitive remediation services to psychiatric patients. She also started an annual conference, *Cognitive Remediation in Psychiatry*, which is cosponsored by several organizations and takes place the first Friday in June. Her groundbreaking research on the role of motivation in learning, and the factors that contribute to effective cognitive remediation with psychiatric populations, has influenced the way cognitive remediation is delivered throughout the world. Dr. Medalia can be reached at amedalia@aol.com.

Nadine Revheim, PhD, is a Research Scientist–Psychologist in the Program of Cognitive Neuroscience and Schizophrenia at the Nathan Kline Institute for Psychiatric Research in Orangeburg, NY, with over 20 years of prior experience as a mental health occupational therapist. After completing her Kessel Fellowship with Dr. Alice Medalia, she continued to investigate cognitive remediation strategies, including those related to the evaluation and treatment of early sensory processing and reading deficits in schizophrenia. She advocates for people with serious mental illness within Rockland County, NY, as a member of NAMI-Family and the Mental Health Coalition, and also has a private practice. Additional research interests include spirituality and coping with psychiatric illness. Dr. Revheim can be reached at nrevheim@aol.com.

Tiffany Herlands, PsyD, is Assistant Professor of Psychiatry and Director of Rehabilitation Psychology at Columbia Presbyterian Eastside. Dr. Herlands has been running Learning Centers since her Kessel Fellowship with Dr. Alice Medalia, and she is a frequent speaker on the topic of treating cognitive disorders. She is the Program Manager for the Lieber Recovery Clinic at Columbia Presbyterian Eastside and trains interested professionals in the design and operation of cognitive remediation programs. Dr. Herlands is also trained in general neuropsychology and works with neurologic populations who present with cognitive impairment. Dr. Herlands can be reached at therlands@aol.com.